Therapeutic uses of cannabis

British Medical Association

harwood academic publishers
Australia • Canada • China • France • Germany • India
Japan • Luxembourg • Malaysia • The Netherlands • Russia
Singapore • Switzerland • Thailand • United Kingdom

1997

Published under licence in The Netherlands under the Harwood Academic Publishers imprint, part of The Gordon and Breach Publishing Group.

 Printed in the United Kingdom.

Amsteldijk 166
1st Floor
1079 LH Amsterdam
The Netherlands

The British Medical Association has published this report in the interests of furthering the clinical and scientific understanding of the potential therapeutic uses of cannabis and cannabinoids. The BMA believes that there should be changes in the law to permit the use of cannabinoids where clinically appropriate under medical supervision.

British Library Cataloguing in Publication Data
A catalogue record for this book is available from the British Library.

ISBN 90-5702-318-0 (soft cover)

Cover photograph: Science Photo Library

Therapeutic uses of cannabis

Contents

3 Therapeutic uses 21

Editorial Board

Board of Science and Education

This report was prepared under the auspices of the Board of Science and Education of the British Medical Association. The members of the Board were as follows:

Sir Donald Acheson	President, BMA
Dr S J Richards	Chairman of the Representative Body, BMA
Dr A W Macara	Chairman of Council, BMA
Dr W J Appleyard	Treasurer, BMA
Professor J B L Howell	Chairman, Board of Science and Education
Dr P Dangerfield	Deputy Chairman, Board of Science and Education
Dr J M Cundy	
Dr H W K Fell	
Miss C E Fozzard	
Dr E Harris	
Dr N J Olsen	
Ms S Somjee	
Dr P Steadman	
Dr S Taylor	
Dr D Ward	

Acknowledgements

The Association is indebted to the following individuals and organizations for their kind permission to reproduce pictures and text in this publication:

Academic Press
American Academy of Ophthalmology
American Association for the Advancement for Science
BMJ Publishing Group
Ms Clare Hodges
CRC Press
Elsevier Science Inc
Galen Press
The Haworth Press
The Lancet Ltd
Lippincott-Raven Publishers
National Academy Press
Springer-Verlag GmbH & Co. KG.
US Cancer Pain Relief Committee
Yale University Press

The Association is grateful for the specialist help provided by the BMA Committees and many outside experts and organizations, and would particularly like to thank:

Action Against Drugs Unit, Home Office; the BMA's Working Party on the Misuse of Drugs; Dr David Bowsher, Research Director, Pain Research Institute, Walton Hospital; Mr Tony Chester; the Drivers Medical Unit, Driver and Vehicle Licensing Agency; Dr Clive Edwards, Senior Lecturer in Clinical Pharmacy, University of Newcastle; Ms Clare Hodges, Alliance for Cannabis Therapeutics; Dr Jeff Kipling, Director of Science and Technology, Association of the British Pharmaceutical Industry; Dr William G Notcutt, Consultant in Anaesthesia and Pain Relief, James Paget Hospital; Mr Mario Price, Senior Pharmacist, James Paget Hospital.

List of tables

List of figures

1

Introduction

The British Medical Association (BMA) is the professional organisation representing the medical professional in the UK. It was established in 1832 'to promote the medical and allied sciences, and to maintain the honour and interests of the profession'. The Board of Science and Education, a standing committee of the Association, supports this aim by acting as an interface between the profession, the government and the public. Its main role is to analyse and review critically issues of interest to the medical profession and the public and to contribute to the improvement of public health. Through this work the BMA has developed policies on a wide range of health issues, such as alcohol, smoking, infectious diseases, complementary medicine, pesticides, and transport safety.

In 1994 the BMA's Annual Representative Meeting (ARM) adopted a resolution, requesting that the Board of Science and Education:

i) *Prepare an authoritative statement on the relative risks of drugs of addiction including the principal controlled drugs, tobacco and alcohol;*

ii) *Advise on the role of the medical profession in relation to:*

a) *drug misusers who wish to discontinue their habit;*

b) *drug misusers who wish to continue their habit;*

c) *arrangements which exist, or might exist in the future, for supplying drugs to either of the above categories of drug misuser;*

iii) *Consider the benefits or otherwise of decriminalization or legalization of some or all controlled drugs.*

The BMA published its report on drug misuse in 1997 (BMA, 1997) addressing parts *i)* and *ii)* of the ARM resolution. In considering part *iii)* of the resolution, the BMA felt that questions regarding the legalization or decriminalization of controlled drugs should be considered only with regard to their therapeutic use by patients under medical supervision, for particular medical conditions. As a subject of wide public and professional interest, the potential therapeutic benefits of cannabis and cannabinoids have therefore been reviewed and are published here as a separate policy document.

In 1997 the BMA's Annual Representative Meeting resolved *That this Representative Body believes that certain additional cannabinoids should be legalized for wider medicinal use*. This report supports and develops this policy statement by describing the scientific evidence for wider medicinal use of cannabinoids and defining future research needs.

The Royal Pharmaceutical Society of Great Britain also believes that action is needed. The Society has called for further clinical research into the potential therapeutic uses of cannabinoids, and while this is underway, that doctors should be able to prescribe cannabinoids for specific serious disorders, at least for a trial period.

Cannabis sativa

The plant *Cannabis sativa*, from which cannabis is obtained, has a long history as a medicine. Over the centuries, its uses have included the treatment of pain, asthma and dysentery, the promotion of sleep, the suppression of nausea and vomiting and the abolition of convulsions and spasms (Mechoulam, 1986). In this country, the medicinal use of cannabis was particularly prominent in the nineteenth century. However, it remained permissible for British doctors to prescribe cannabis (as a tincture for oral administration) until 1971. More recently, claims have been made for the beneficial effects of cannabis and cannabinoids (a family of carbon, hydrogen and oxygen containing compounds which constitute the active ingredients of cannabis). This interest has coincided with a renewed interest in and increasing acceptance of herbal medicine and 'natural' remedies.

The legal situation

Cannabis and certain psychoactive cannabinoids and derivatives (cannabinol and its derivatives tetrahydrocannabinol and 3-alkyl homologues of cannabinol or its tetra hydro derivatives) are classified under Schedule 1 of the Misuse of Drugs Act 1971 as having no therapeutic benefit. They therefore cannot be prescribed by doctors or dispensed by pharmacists and can only be possessed for research purposes with a Home Office licence. If the research involves clinical trials, further permission is required from the Medicines Control Agency.

Two other non-psychoactive cannabinoids, cannabidiol and cannabichromene, despite their structural similarity to cannabinol, are not controlled drugs; although not licensed as medicines, there is nothing to prevent a doctor from prescribing them. A further two cannabinoids, dronabinol and nabilone, can be prescribed by doctors.

Nabilone, a synthetic analogue of Δ^9-tetrahydrocannabinol (THC), is licensed for prescription to patients with nausea or vomiting resulting from cancer chemotherapy which has proved unresponsive to other drugs. A change in international law has allowed the prescription of Δ^9-THC (dronabinol) for the same indication. Following advice from the World Health Organization to the United Nations Commission on Narcotic Drugs that dronabinol had demonstrated medical uses in combatting nausea and vomiting caused by cancer chemotherapy, the United Nations Commission on Narcotic Drugs rescheduled dronabinol under the UN Convention on Psychotropic Substances 1971. This in turn led the UK Government, a signatory to the UN Convention, to reschedule dronabinol from Schedule 1 to Schedule 2 under the Misuse of Drugs Act. Dronabinol is currently unlicensed in the UK and has to be specially imported for prescription on a 'named patient basis' for the same indication. Prescribing unlicensed medicines puts greater responsibility on the doctor, as their effects may be less well understood than those of licensed products.

International developments

In 1996 in the United States, Arizona passed a law permitting doctors to prescribe any drug in Schedule I (which are not approved by the Food and Drug Administration) including cannabis, but this was effectively repealed by the FDA the following year. In the same year Californian voters approved a state law eliminating criminal penalties for those who grew or used small amounts of cannabis for medical purposes if they could show that they were acting on the recommendation of a doctor. However, under federal law, cannabis remains an illegal narcotic, and doctors who recommend its use to patients have been threatened with prosecution and loss of their prescription privileges under Drug Enforcement Administration regulations.

In Italy patients who need cannabis for therapeutic purposes are allowed to grow their own supply of the plant once they have gained certification from their local authority and in Germany nabilone is unlicensed but can be imported for prescription.

Until August 1997, doctors in the Netherlands were able, unofficially, to issue prescriptions for cannabis which were dispensed by pharmacists. However, acting on a recent report by the Dutch Health Council (1996) which concluded that there was insufficient proof of its medicinal benefits, the health inspectorate has banned the prescription of cannabis. It remains available from 'brown' coffee shops, but is of unregulated quality. In most other European countries cannabis and cannabinoids remain illegal for therapeutic use.

Prescription of unlicensed medicines in the UK *(Drug and therapeutics bulletin, 1992)*

As an unlicensed medicine, the prescription of dronabinol or of nabilone for an unlicensed indication, brings with it extra responsibilities for the doctor. The legal responsibility for prescribing any medicine lies with the doctor, for an unlicensed medicine, or for an unlicensed indication, (one which is not on the data sheet) the prescriber can be particularly vulnerable. In common law doctors have a duty to take reasonable care and act in a way consistent with the practice of a responsible body of their peers of similar professional standing. Not to meet this standard would lay the doctor open to allegations of negligence.

When prescribing outside a licence, it is important that doctors should do so knowingly; where possible, the drug's licence status should be explained to patients in sufficient details to allow them to give informed consent. This will involve explaining that the effects of an unlicensed product may be less well understood than those of a licensed product. Prescribers need to be fully informed about the uses and actions of the product and assured of its quality and source.

Scope and purpose of the report

This report provides an outline of the pharmacology of cannabis and cannabinoids relevant to medicinal aspects, followed by short reviews of the main proposed therapeutic uses. These reviews are presented as follows:

- Suggested therapeutic indication and its medical importance.
- Existing pharmacological treatments and their shortcomings.
- Human studies on the use of cannabis/cannabinoids in the condition under discussion.
- Further research needed.
- Conclusion and recommendations.

The literature covered is not claimed to be exhaustive, but it is believed to be sufficiently comprehensive to provide an overall picture of the area reviewed. In many areas definite conclusions are not possible because of the absence of data. In such cases the type of data required is suggested. A glossary of terms used in this report is given in Appendix I.

2

Pharmacology

Constituents of cannabis; natural and synthetic cannabinoids

Cannabis sativa and some of its subspecies contain over 400 chemical compounds amongst which more than 60 cannabinoids (chemicals unique to the genus *Cannabis*) have been identified.[1] The pharmacology of many of these constituents is unknown but the most potent psychoactive agent, delta-9-tetrahydrocannabinol (Δ^9-THC, referred to in this review as THC), has been isolated, synthesised and much studied. THC is not only the main psychoactive agent but is also responsible for many of the other pharmacological actions of cannabis. Other natural cannabinoids are delta-8-tetrahydrocannabinol (Δ^8-THC), cannabinol, and cannabidiol (Fig. 1). In addition, several synthetic cannabinoids are available (Fig. 2 and Table 1). Some properties of various cannabinoids are outlined in Table 1. For medicinal purposes, the synthetic cannabinoid nabilone is licensed for medicinal use in this country, and dronabinol (synthetic THC in sesame oil) is licensed

1 Throughout this report the monoterpinoid numbering system for chemical compounds is used. The older pyran system is not generally applicable since some cannabinoids are not pyrans. For further explanation see Mechoulam R, (1973) Marijuana - Chemistry, Pharmacology, metabolism and clinical effects. Academic Press

Figure 1: Chemical structure of main cannabinoids in *Cannabis sativa* (Maykut, 1985)

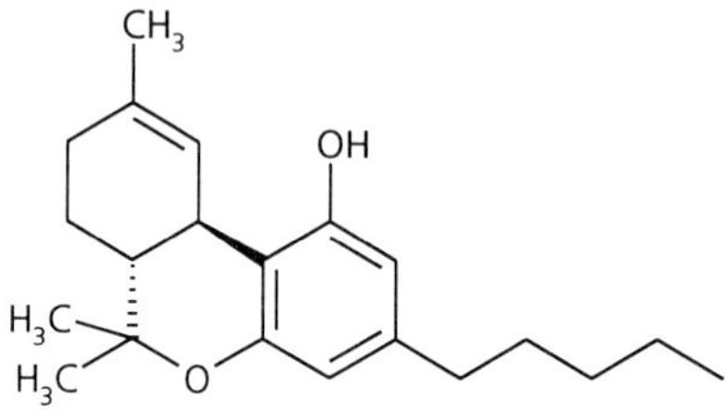

Δ^9-Tetrahydrocannabinol (Δ^9-THC)

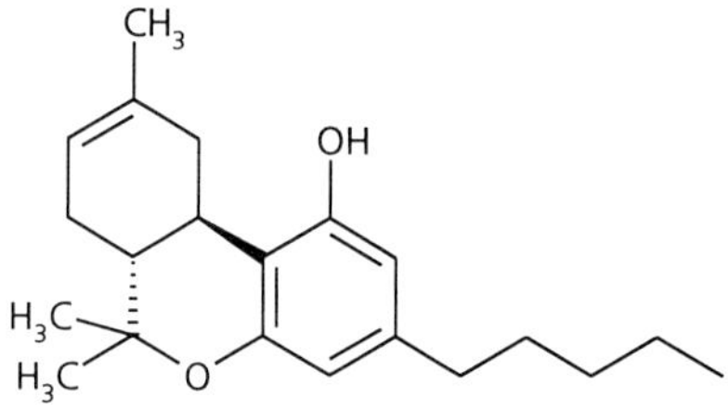

Δ^8-Tetrahydrocannabinol (Δ^8-THC)

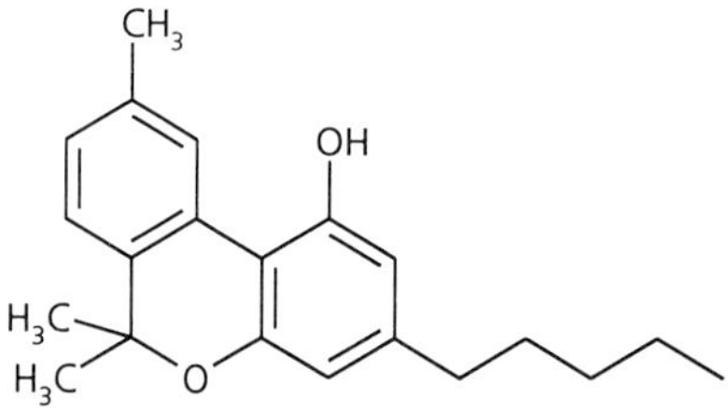

Cannabinol (CBN)

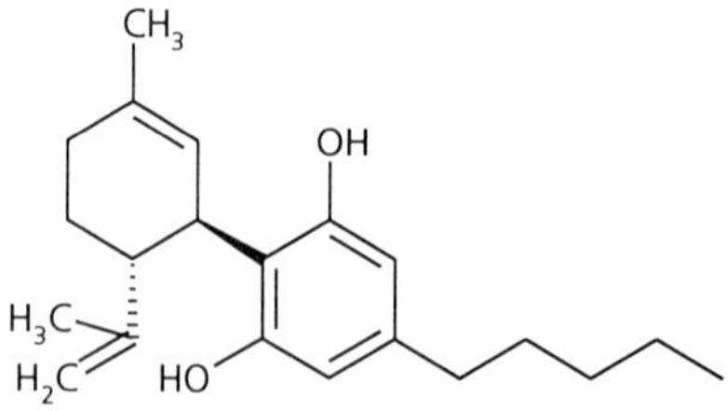

Cannabidiol (CBD)

Figure 2: Structure of some synthetic cannabinoids and anandamide (Consroe and Sandyk, 1992; Pertwee 1995)

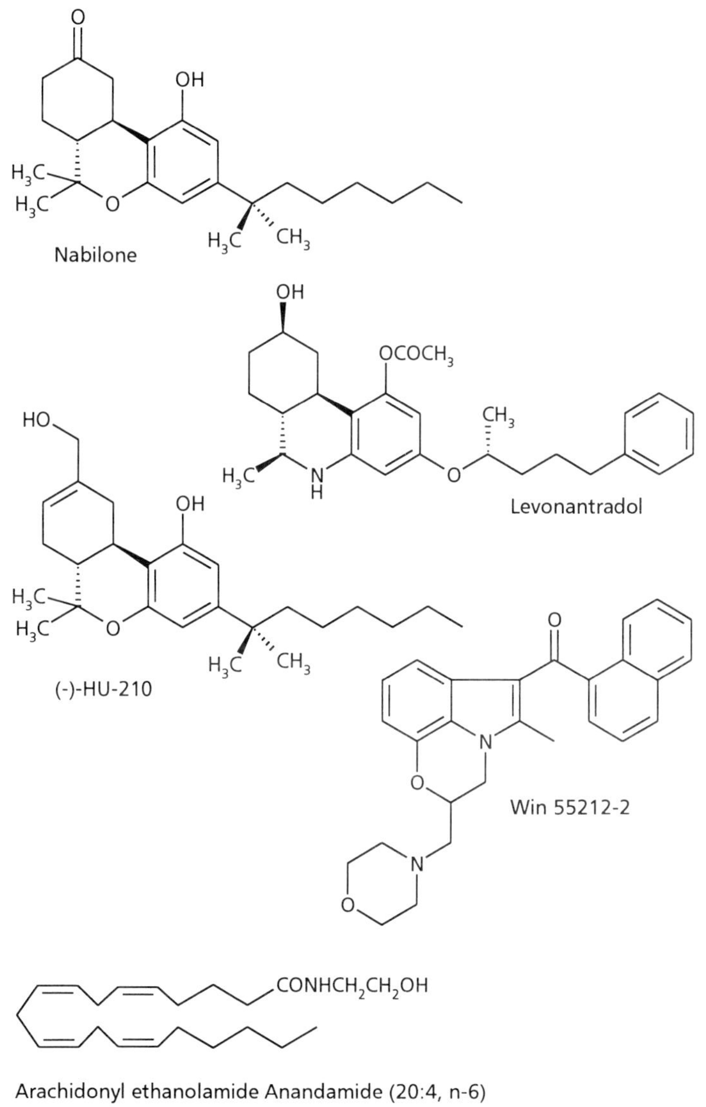

for use in the USA. Other compounds in the smoke from cannabis preparations, including carbon monoxide, tars, irritants and carcinogens, are similar to those in tobacco smoke (Table 2).

Table 1: Properties of some natural and synthetic cannabinoids *(see Figs. 1 and 2 for chemical structures)*

The data given in this table refers to research on both animals and humans. All references to psychoactive/lack of psychoactive effects refer to humans. All references to binding to cannabis receptors refer to animal work. The last four synthetic compounds (-)-HU-210, (+)-HU-210, Win55212-2 and SR141716A have only been studied in animals.

Δ^9-tetrahydrocannabinol (Δ^9-THC) Natural plant cannabinoid Available in synthetic form as dronabinol (THC in sesame oil)	Main psychoactive cannabinoid in *Cannabis sativa*; largely responsible for psychological and physical effects.
Δ^8-tetrahydrocannabinol (Δ^8-THC) Natural plant cannabinoid Also available in synthetic form	Slightly less potent than Δ^9-THC but otherwise similar. Only small amounts present in plant. Appears to have few psychoactive effects in children.
Cannabinol Natural plant cannabinoid	Less potent than Δ^9-THC.
Cannabidiol Natural plant cannabinoid	Does not interact with cannabinoid receptors. Lacks psychotropic and most other effects of Δ^9-THC, but has anticonvulsant activity and may have analgesic properties. May attenuate some unwanted psychological effects of THC.
Cannabichromene Natural plant cannabinoid	Does not interact with cannabinoid receptors. Not psychoactive but may enhance some effects of THC.
11-hydroxy-Δ^9-THC Natural metabolite of Δ^9-THC in the body	Psychoactive; may be responsible for some of the psychological effects of cannabis.
(-)-Δ^8-THC-11-oic acid Natural metabolite of Δ^8-THC in the body	Does not interact with cannabinoid receptors; not psychoactive but has analgesic activity.

Anandamide (arachidonyl ethanolamide) Endogenous ligand for mammalian cannabinoid receptors	Not structurally similar to cannabinoids; related to prostaglandins. Appears to mimic actions of THC and other cannabinoids that interact with cannabinoid receptors.
Nabilone Synthetic cannabinoid	Similar pharmacological properties to THC but more potent. Possibly more likely to produce dysphoria than THC, but lower incidence of euphoria and less abuse potential.
Levonantradol Synthetic cannabinoid	Pharmacological properties similar to THC, but more potent analgesic effects. High incidence of dysphoria and other side-effects.
(-)-HU-210 Synthetic cannabinoid	Pharmacological properties similar to levonantradol.
(+)-HU-210 Synthetic cannabinoid (stereoisomer of (-)-HU-210)	Does not interact with cannabinoid receptors but appears to be an antagonist of NMDA*, giving it a potential for use in stroke and neurodegenerative disorders.
Win 55212-2 Synthetic compound	Different chemical structure to known cannabinoids but binds to cannabis receptors. Similar compounds may act as cannabinoid antagonists - important for further understanding of the physiological and therapeutic role of cannabinoids.
SR 141716 A Synthetic compound	Cannabis CB_1 receptor antagonist

*NMDA - N-methyl-D-aspartate, an important excitatory neurotransmitter in the brain, involved in learning and memory, epilepsy, strokes, and neurodegenerative disorders.
References: Maykut, 1985; Consroe and Sandyk, 1992; Pertwee, 1995.

Pharmacokinetics

This section draws on the reviews carried out by Agurell et al., 1986; Maykut, 1985; Gold, 1992, and others.

Absorption

THC and other cannabinoids are rapidly absorbed on inhalation from smoked cannabis preparations. The amount absorbed depends on smoking style but may be 20-45% of the THC content of a cannabis cigarette. Effects are perceptible within seconds and become fully apparent in a matter of minutes. When taken orally absorption of THC is variable and much slower. Blood concentrations reached are 25-30% of those obtained by smoking the same dose, partly due to the fact that some of the THC is degraded by metabolism in the liver before reaching the circulation (first-pass metabolism) although the metabolite 11-hydroxy-Δ^9-THC is also psychoactive. The onset of effect is delayed (0.5-2 hours) but the duration of effect may be prolonged due to continual slow absorption from the gut.

Because of their insolubility in water, it has been difficult to formulate preparations of pure cannabinoids for medicinal use. However dronabinol (synthetic THC in sesame oil) is suitable for oral use (see Nausea and vomiting associated with cancer chemotherapy p.21-23). Other methods of administration which have been used experimentally or therapeutically with varying success include aerosols and sprays (see Bronchial asthma, p.59-63), eye drops (see Glaucoma, p.53-59), and rectal administration which avoids first-pass metabolism (see Dosage and routes of administration, p.73-74). Intravenous administration requires dissolving THC in alcohol and delivering in a fast-flowing saline infusion, a method not practical for general medical use.

Distribution *(Figure 3)*

After smoking or intravenous administration, THC and other cannabinoids are rapidly distributed throughout the body reaching first the tissues with the highest blood flow (brain, lungs, liver, adrenals, kidney, ovaries and testes). Maximum brain

Figure 3: Distribution of THC in the body. Graph from Nahas GG. (1975) after Kreutz and Axelrod (1973)

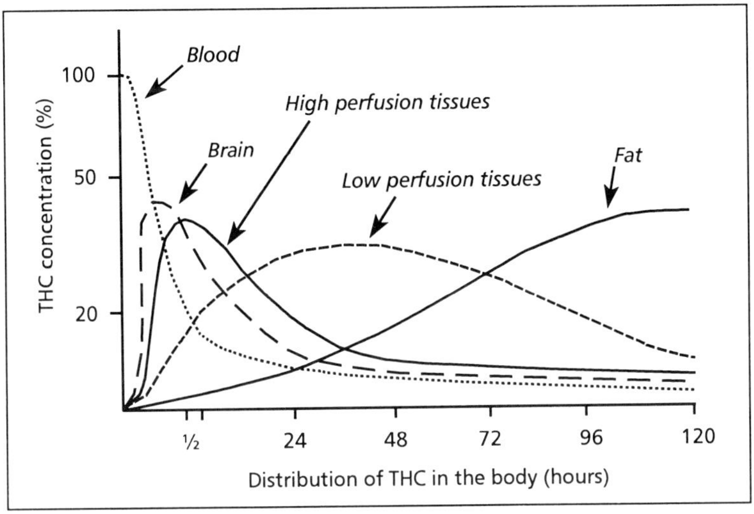

concentrations are reached within 15 minutes, coinciding with the onset of maximal psychological and physiological effects. The psychological effects then reach a plateau which can last for several hours (2-4), before slowly declining. Heart rate changes decline much faster as THC leaves the bloodstream and enters the brain.

After oral administration maximal effects occur after an hour or more but may last 5-6 hours because of continued absorption from the gut, but some psychomotor and cognitive effects persist for much longer (Leirer et al., 1991), probably for more than 24 hours, regardless of the mode of administration. Cannabinoids also cross the placenta, enter the foetal circulation, and penetrate into breast milk.

Cannabinoids are highly lipid soluble and accumulate in fatty tissues, from which they are only slowly released back into other body tissues and organs, including the bloodstream and the brain. Because of this sequestration in fat, elimination from the body is extremely slow but although complete elimination of a single dose can take up to 30 days (Maykut, 1985), the therapeutic concentration would last a much shorter time. Clearly, with repeated dosage cannabinoids can accumulate in the body and continue to reach the brain over a longer period.

Table 2: Constituents of mainstream smoke in cannabis and tobacco cigarettes

Measurements	**Marihuana Cigarette (85mm)**	**Tobacco Cigarette (85mm)**
Cigarettes Average weight, mg	1,115.0	1,110.0
Moisture, %	10.3	11.1
Pressure drop, cm	14.7	7.2
Static burning rate, mg/s	0.88	0.80
Puff number	10.7	11.1
Mainstream smoke **Gas phase** Carbon monoxide, vol. %	3.99	4.58
mg	17.6	20.2
Carbon dioxide, vol. %	8.27	9.38
mg	57.3	65.0
Ammonia, µg	228.0	199.0
HCN, µg	532.0	498.0
Cyanogen $(CN)_2$, µg	19.0	20.0
Isoprene, µg	83.0	310.0
Acetaldehyde, µg	1,200.0	980.0
Acetone, µg	443.0	578.0
Acrolein, µg	92.0	85.0
Acetonitrile, µg	132.0	123.0
Benzene, µg	76.0	67.0
Toluene, µg	112.0	108.0
Vinyl chloride ng*	5.4	12.4
Dimethylnitrosamine,ng*	75.0	84.0
Methylethylnitrosamine,ng*	27.0	30.0

pH, third puff	6.56	6.14
fifth puff	6.57	6.15
seventh puff	6.58	6.14
ninth puff	6.56	6.10
tenth puff	6.58	6.02
Particulate phase Total particulate matter, dry, mg	22.7	39.0
Phenol, µg	76.8	138.5
o-Cresol, µg	17.9	24.0
m- and *p*-Cresol, µg	54.4	65.0
Dimethylphenol, µg	6.8	14.4
Catechol, µg	188.0	328.0
Cannabidiol, µg	190.0	-
delta^9-Tetrahydrocannabinol, µg	820.0	-
Cannabinol, µg	400.0	-
Nicotine, µg	-	2,850.0
N-Nitrosonornicotine, ng*	-	390.0
Naphthalene, µg	3.0	1.2
1-Methylnaphthalene, µg	6.1	3.65
2-Methylnaphthalene, µg	3.6	1.4
Benz(a)anthracene, ng*	75.0	43.0
Benzo(a)pyrene, ng*	31.0	21.1

* Indicates known carcinogens.

From *Marihuana and Health*, p16, National Academy of Sciences, Institute of Medicine Report, Washington D.C., 1982. It should be noted that there may be additives in illegally obtained cannabis, either from the agricultural process eg pesticides or packing materials. Such additives may change the composition of the smoke.

Metabolism and excretion

Cannabinoids are metabolised in the liver. A major metabolite is 11-hydroxy-Δ^9-THC (Table 1) which is possibly more potent than Δ^9-THC itself, and may be responsible for some of the psychological and physiological effects of cannabis. More than 20 other metabolites are known, some of which may also be psychoactive. These metabolites are slowly excreted, over days or weeks, in the urine and faeces. There are large interindividual differences in rates of metabolism, and metabolism is likely to be slowed in the elderly and in the presence of liver disease.

Pharmacodynamics

Understanding of the pharmacodynamics of cannabinoids has been greatly enhanced recently by the discovery and cloning of specific cannabinoid receptors in the mammalian brain (Devane et al., 1988; Matsuda et al., 1990) and human brain and spleen (Munro et al., 1993), and the identification of natural (endogenous) substances which bind to these receptors (Devane et al., 1992; Pertwee, 1995). There appears to be a natural cannabinoid receptor-neuromodulator system in the body through which cannabinoids exert their effects. Recent advances in this field are reviewed by Howlett et al. (1990), Herkenham et al. (1995), Deadwyler et al. (1995), Pertwee (1995), and Musty et al. (1995), among others.

Cannabinoid receptors

Cannabinoid receptors in the brain, CB_1 receptors, are distributed in discrete areas including those concerned with motor activity and postural control (basal ganglia, cerebellum), memory and cognition (cerebral cortex and hippocampus), emotion (amygdala and hippocampus), sensory perception (thalamus), and autonomic and endocrine functions (hypothalamus, pons, medulla). The distribution of cannabinoid receptors is similar to the distribution of injected THC and other cannabinoids; these compounds undoubtedly exert many of their pharmacological effects by interaction with these receptors. A second type of cannabinoid receptor, the CB_2 receptor, has been detected in the macrophages (immune cells) of the spleen and probably mediates the immunological effects of cannabinoids.

While CB_1 receptors are found in the central nervous system, both CB_1 and CB_2 receptors are present in peripheral tissues. Cannabinoids, such as THC, which activate the central CB_1 receptors are psychoactive. A major implication of the discovery of cannabinoid receptors is that it should be possible to develop selective cannabinoid agonists and antagonists for use either as therapeutic agents or as experimental tools to help establish physiological roles of cannabinoid receptors and endogenous compounds which bind to these receptors (e.g. the anandamides).

Endogenous cannabinoids — anandamide and others

The first endogenous substance which was shown to interact specifically with cannabinoid receptors was christened anandamide after the Sanskrit word for bliss, "ananda". It has a different chemical structure from plant-derived and synthetic cannabinoids (Fig. 2) being a derivative of the endogenous fatty acid arachidonic acid (arachidonyl ethanolamide). Two similar endogenous fatty acid derivatives have since been isolated. In animals these compounds exert many of the actions of THC (they have not been tested in man). However, it now appears that the mammalian body contains a whole system of, perhaps multiple, cannabinoid receptors and anandamide-related substances.

Mechanism of action

Despite this new knowledge, the mechanisms of action and the physiological functions of this system remain obscure. Present information suggests that both cannabinoid receptors and anandamides reside within neuronal membranes. Unlike classical neurotransmitters such as noradrenaline and acetylcholine, anandamides are not released into extracellular spaces and are not involved in interneuronal communication. Instead the system appears to modulate the excitability and responsiveness of neurones by influencing intraneuronal events such as the formation of cyclic AMP (adenosine monophosphate, energy-providing compound) and the transport of calcium and potassium ions (necessary for excitation) across the nerve membranes. In this covert role, the cannabinoid-anandamide system undoubtedly interacts with many other neurotransmitter/neuromodulator systems including cholinergic, noradrenergic, dopaminergic, serotonergic, GABA (gamma-amino-butyric acid), NMDA (N-methyl-D-aspartate), opioid, glucocorticoid, and prostaglandin systems. All of these interactions are under investigation but their role in the pharmacological effects of cannabinoids are not yet clear.

Until this system is unravelled it remains impossible to explain adequately the mechanisms of action of exogenously administered cannabinoids. However, it is clear that cannabinoids join the many other classes of drugs, such as opioids and benzodiazepines, whose pharmacological actions result from their inadvertent entrance into, and perturbation of, endogenous neuromodulatory systems.

Actions of cannabis in man *(Table 3)*

Cannabinoids affect almost every body system. Their effects have been reviewed by Paton and Pertwee (1973), Nahas (1984), Maykut (1985), Hollister (1986, 1988), Mendelson (1987), Gold (1991, 1992) and many others. A full description of these effects is beyond the scope of this review but the main actions are summarised in Table 3. Many of these actions are unwanted in the therapeutic setting, as discussed in Section 4.

Table 3: Some pharmacological actions of cannabis in man (in therapeutic dosage range)

Central nervous system Psychological effects	Euphoria ("high"), dysphoria, anxiety, depersonalisation, precipitation/aggravation of psychotic states.
Effects on perception	Heightened sensory perception, distortion of space and time sense, misperceptions, hallucinations.
Sedative effects	Generalised CNS depression, drowsiness, sleep, additive effects with other CNS depressants.
Effects on cognition and psychomotor performance	Fragmentation of thoughts, mental clouding, memory impairment, global impairment of performance especially in complex and demanding tasks.
Effects on motor function	Increased motor activity followed by inertia and incoordination, ataxia, dysarthria, tremulousness, weakness, muscle twitching.
Analgesic effects	Similar in potency to codeine (but by a non-opioid mechanism).
Anti-emetic effects Increased appetite	In acute doses; effect reversed with larger doses or chronic use.
Tolerance	To most behavioural and somatic effects, including the "high" with chronic use.
Dependence, abstinence syndrome	Rarely observed but has been produced experimentally following prolonged intoxication: symptoms include disturbed sleep, decreased appetite, restlessness, irritability and sweating.
Cardiovascular system Heart rate	Tachycardia with acute dosage; bradycardia with chronic use.
Peripheral circulation	Vasodilatation, conjunctival redness, postural hypotension.
Cardiac output	Increased output and myocardial oxygen demand.
Cerebral blood flow	Increased acutely, decreased with chronic use.
Respiratory system Ventilation	Small doses stimulate, larger doses depress.
Bronchodilatation	Coughing, but tolerance develops.
Airways obstruction	Chronic smoking.
Eye	Decreased intraocular pressure.
Immune system	Impaired bacteriocidal activity of macrophages in lung and spleen (chronic use).

Reproductive system	
Males	Antiandrogenic, decreased sperm count and sperm motility (chronic use).
Females	Suppression of ovulation, complex effects on prolactin secretion, increased obstetric risks (chronic use).

Note: Many of the effects are biphasic, e.g. increased activity with acute or smaller doses, decreased activity with larger doses or chronic use. Effects vary greatly between individuals and may be greater in elderly or ill patients.

Of relevance to the therapeutic use of cannabinoids are the antiemetic, muscle relaxant, analgesic, anti-inflammatory, appetite stimulant, anticonvulsant and bronchodilator effects and the effects on intraocular pressure. All these effects are discussed in the following sections on potential therapeutic uses. It should be stressed that the mechanism of none of these actions is fully understood. There are plenty of hints and speculations but, in the interests of brevity and because they remain uncertain, possible mechanisms of action are not discussed in this report. Referring to the best known and accepted therapeutic use of cannabinoids as anti-emetics, Levitt (1986) comments:

> *"The use of cannabinoids as cancer chemotherapy anti-emetics represents, in essence, the use of a drug with a relatively undefined mechanism of action to treat the side-effects of other drugs, also with relatively undefined mechanisms of action, which are being used to treat cancer, a disease or series of diseases the precise nature of which remains enigmatic."*
>
> (Levitt, 1986, p.77)

With this level of ignorance in mind, the available evidence on the therapeutic potential of cannabinoids is reviewed below.

3

Therapeutic uses

Nausea and vomiting associated with cancer chemotherapy

One of the most distressing symptoms in medicine is the prolonged nausea and vomiting which regularly accompanies treatment with many anti-cancer agents. This can be so severe that patients come to dread their treatment; some find the side-effects of the drugs worse than the disease they are designed to treat; others find the symptoms so intolerable that they decline further therapy despite the presence of malignant disease. With some anti-cancer agents (notably mustine, dacarbazine, cisplatin, cyclophosphamide, doxorubicin and high dose methotrexate) nausea and vomiting is so common that anti-emetic drugs are routinely given before and after treatment. One of these is the synthetic cannabinoid nabilone, which is the only cannabinoid licensed for use in the UK; dronabinol (synthetic THC in sesame oil) is also licensed in the USA and can be prescribed for this indication on a named patient basis in the UK.

Existing pharmacological treatments

Phenothiazines (e.g. prochlorperazine, haloperidol) are dopamine receptor antagonists and act by blocking the chemoreceptor trigger zone, part of the vomiting centre in the brain. They are generally effective but have numerous side-effects including severe dystonic reactions, especially in children and elderly or debilitated patients. Other effects include drowsiness, dry mouth, blurred vision, urinary retention, hypotension, allergic reactions, and occasionally jaundice.

Metoclopramide is also a dopamine receptor antagonist and has actions similar to phenothiazines. It can induce acute dystonic reactions with facial and skeletal muscle spasms, especially in the young and the very old. Other side-effects include drowsiness, restlessness, diarrhoea, and depression.

Domperidone is another dopamine receptor antagonist which acts at the chemoreceptor trigger zone. It does not readily enter the rest of the brain and is less likely to cause sedation although it can cause acute dystonic reactions.

Selective serotonin 5-HT$_3$ receptor antagonists (e.g. ondansetron, granisetron) have been licensed relatively recently. They appear to be valuable for patients in whom other anti- emetics are ineffective or not tolerated. Reported side-effects include constipation, headache and alterations in liver function. These drugs are expensive. They can be given by mouth but intravenous infusion may be required in patients treated by anti-cancer agents which produce severe vomiting.

Nabilone is a synthetic cannabinoid with proved anti-emetic effects though the mode of action is unknown. Side-effects occur in most patients given standard doses and include drowsiness, euphoria or dysphoria, concentration difficulty, ataxia, visual disturbance, dry mouth, hypotension. Confusion, disorientation, hallucinations, psychosis and tremor are also reported. Nabilone is licensed for hospital use only for the sole indication "nausea and vomiting caused by cytotoxic chemotherapy, unresponsive to conventional anti-emetics" (British National Formulary,

September 1996). It is not recommended for patients under 18 years of age.

Adjuvant treatments. For chemotherapeutic agents that produce moderate or severe vomiting a corticosteroid (dexamethasone) and a benzodiazepine tranquilliser (lorazepam) are usually given in addition to anti-emetic drugs, before and after chemotherapy.

All these drugs are moderately though not completely effective. Dystonic reactions as well as other side-effects are a major disadvantage with dopamine receptor antagonists. Selective serotonin antagonists look promising but their place has not been fully evaluated. Nabilone is also effective but is also not without unwanted effects. There is a need for a non-toxic anti-emetic suitable for use at all ages, which does not cause dystonic reactions or undue sedation.

Cannabis and cannabinoids in vomiting due to anti-cancer drugs *(Tables i and ii)*

Of all the potential medicinal uses of cannabinoids, there is most information on their effects in nausea and vomiting caused by anti-cancer drugs. A comprehensive review of the literature is not given here but the results from a selection of 23 well-controlled trials of THC and nabilone are summarised in Tables i and ii. A review by Levitt (1986) cites 55 studies, 32 of which were of randomised double-blind design; other reviews (Vincent et al., 1983; Formukong et al, 1989) describe further studies. The overwhelming conclusion from controlled trials is that both THC and nabilone can be effective anti-emetics in patients receiving anti-neoplastic agents. Some studies suggest that cannabinoids are more effective than standard drugs including prochlorperazine, metoclopramide and domperidone (Nagy et al., 1978; Herman et al., 1979; Einhorn et al., 1981; Niiranen and Mattson, 1985;

Niederle et al., 1986; Pomeroy et al., 1986; Dalzell et al., 1986; Chan et al., 1987; Orr and McKernan, 1981; Lucas et al., 1980). Other studies found cannabinoids were of equal effectiveness to standard drugs (Frytak et al., 1979; Niedhart et al., 1981; Ungerleider et al., 1982). Relatively few studies have found THC to be less effective than standard drugs or placebo (Chang et al., 1981; Gralla et al., 1982; Lane et al., 1991). The combination of THC and prochlorperazine appeared to be more effective than either drug given alone (Lane et al., 1990, 1991), and nabilone combined with prochlorperazine was found to be better than metoclopramide combined with dexamethasone (Cunningham et al., 1988). Plasse et al. (1991) comment that prochlorperazine may counteract the dysphoric effects of THC to some extent.

Most investigations have found that the side-effects of both THC and nabilone are greater than those of standard drugs. These commonly include drowsiness, dry mouth, ataxia, visual disturbances and dysphoric reactions. Frytak et al. (1979) reported that such side-effects with THC were sometimes intolerable. On the other hand, in many trials patients (including children) were reported to prefer cannabinoids to standard drugs, despite their greater side-effects.

The synthetic cannabinoid levonantradol has been tested as an anti-emetic in some studies reviewed by Levitt (1986) and Johnson and Melvin (1986), although there have been few controlled trials. The results have been equivocal but the combined evidence suggests that although levonantradol is sometimes effective as an anti-emetic, it produces an unacceptably high incidence of unpleasant adverse effects including somnolence (50-100% incidence) and dysphoria (30-50% incidence). A more positive result was reported in a recent pilot-study of Δ^8-THC compared with metoclopramide in eight children receiving antineoplastic therapy (Abrahamov et al., 1995). Vomiting occurred in 60% of children receiving metoclopramide but Δ^8-THC given orally before and after treatment completely prevented vomiting during treatment and over the following two days. Two children on Δ^8-THC were "slightly irritable" and one showed "slight euphoria". A planned controlled comparison was abandoned on ethical grounds when it became clear that Δ^8-THC was superior to metoclopramide.

Some investigators (Chang et al., 1979) have found smoked cannabis to be more effective than oral THC. This may be because inhaled THC is more readily absorbed than oral THC and also because cannabis contains other substances which enhance the effect of THC. To improve absorption, the use of nasal aerosol or metered inhalers of THC has been recommended (Schwartz and Voth, 1995). In addition to patients undergoing chemotherapy, others, such as those with HIV/AIDS may suffer from nausea and vomiting, sometimes resulting from anti-viral therapy.

Research needed

Cannabinoids are undoubtedly effective as anti-emetics in patients with a variety of cancers being treated by a range of anti-cancer drugs which cause vomiting. The anti-emetic potency of cannabinoids is at least equivalent to that of many widely used anti-emetics. However, there are a number of unanswered questions towards which future research could usefully be directed.

First, cannabinoids have not been compared with the newer specific 5-HT_3 receptor antagonists (ondansetron, granisetron, tropisetron). Such a comparison would be worthwhile to establish the relative efficacy of cannabinoids. It is possible that a combination with cannabinoids might be beneficial and might obviate the need for lengthy intravenous infusions of specific 5-HT_3 antagonists.

Secondly, optimal regimens for administering cannabinoids have not been established, with regard to dosage schedules, timing of administration or combinations with other drugs. Adverse effects of cannabinoids (particularly somnolence and dysphoria) are sometimes limiting factors in clinical use, but it is possible that lower dosages used in combination with other drugs (such as prochlorperazine) might minimise the side effects of the drugs while maximising the therapeutic benefits. In addition, better psychological preparation and explanation to patients may help to limit dysphoric reactions, which are often due to unexpected effects.

Thirdly, it is not clear for which patients or for which types of cancer chemotherapy cannabinoids are most appropriate. Most trials have been carried out on patients with various types of cancer receiving a variety of chemotherapeutic agents. Systematic trials of the effectiveness of cannabinoids in controlling vomiting produced by different agents would be helpful. At present it appears that they may not be helpful for vomiting caused by adriamycin and cyclophosphamide (Chang et al., 1981) but they may be better than other agents for patients on cisplatin and doxorubicin. A clear profile of action would be valuable.

Fourthly, the relative therapeutic efficacy of different cannabinoids has not been established. Both THC and nabilone have been shown to be effective but have not been compared with regard to efficacy or incidence and severity of side-effects. Levonantradol, although effective, appears to have an unacceptable incidence of side-effects, but studies with the less psychoactive Δ^8-THC would be worth pursuing (Abrahamov et al. 1995), and there is a potential for developing new more selectively anti-emetic cannabinoids (Levitt, 1986).

Fifthly, while studies to date have focused on the anti-emetic benefits for patients being treated with anti-cancer drugs, the potential of cannabinoids for severe nausea and vomiting of different origins should be researched.

Finally, the potential immunosuppressive effects of cannabinoids and the consequences for patients who are immunosuppressed as a result of cancer chemotherapy or other conditions need to be established.

Conclusions

- Cannabinoids are undoubtedly effective as anti-emetic agents in vomiting induced by anti-cancer drugs.
- Further research is needed to compare their efficacy with other anti-emetic agents, particularly the relatively newly introduced specific 5-HT_3 antagonists, and optimal routes of administration.
- Further research is needed to establish optimal dosage regimens for cannabinoids, optimal combinations with standard drugs, and specific anti-cancer therapies and types of cancer patients in which they are most beneficial.
- Further research is needed to establish which particular cannabinoids (THC, nabilone, Δ^8-THC or others) have the optimal therapeutic profile as anti-emetics. THC (dronabinol) could usefully be permitted to be prescribed for this indication in the UK.
- Systematic trials of the effectiveness of cannabinoids in combatting vomiting resulting from different chemotherapy agents should be carried out.
- Further research into the immunological effects of cannabinoids is needed to establish their suitability for patients undergoing cancer chemotherapy.

Muscle spasticity

Muscle spasticity, with recurrent painful muscle cramps and various combinations of weakness, tremor, dystonia, abnormal movements, ataxia and decreased bladder and bowel control, occur in a number of chronic and debilitating neurological conditions including multiple sclerosis (MS), cerebral palsy and spinal cord injuries. A variety of drug treatments are available but none are completely satisfactory and there are no effective treatments for tremor, ataxia or muscle weakness.

Existing pharmacological treatments

Muscle relaxants

Baclofen is a GABA (gamma aminobutyric acid) derivative which acts as an agonist at $GABA_B$ receptors, reducing skeletal muscle tone by inhibiting the release of excitatory transmitters mainly at spinal cord level. However, it also affects the brain and can cause many adverse effects. Sedation, drowsiness and nausea are common; lightheadedness, lassitude, confusion, dizziness, ataxia, headaches, depression, hallucinations or euphoria, insomnia, tremor, nystagmus, paraesthesia, convulsions, muscle pain and weakness, respiratory or cardiovascular depression, hypotension, dry mouth, gastrointestinal and urinary disturbances have all been reported occasionally; rarely it can cause visual and taste alterations, sweating, skin rashes, altered blood sugar and liver function and paradoxical increase in spasticity. In addition, a degree of tolerance develops to the muscle relaxant actions and rebound effects occur on withdrawal.

Diazepam and other benzodiazepines act on GABA/benzodiazepine receptors, enhancing the action of GABA at many brain sites and producing muscle relaxation at supraspinal levels. Adverse effects are frequent and include drowsiness, confusion, amnesia, ataxia, paradoxical excitement, tolerance, dependence, and withdrawal effects on discontinuation.

Dantrolene acts directly on skeletal muscle through an effect on intracellular calcium ion release. Adverse effects include drowsiness, dizziness, weakness, malaise, fatigue, diarrhoea, anorexia, nausea, headache, skin rashes. Less frequent are constipation, dysphagia, speech and visual disturbances, confusion, nervousness, insomnia, depression, seizures, chills, fever, urinary frequency. Rarely reported are tachycardia, blood pressure fluctuations, dyspnoea, urinary difficulties, and liver damage. It is necessary to monitor liver function during treatment, and the drug should be used with caution if cardiac or pulmonary function is impaired.

It is clear that these drugs have major limitations. Apart from their many other adverse effects, all have a tendency to aggravate muscle weakness and may worsen the ability to walk in many patients who rely on spasticity or extensor spasms for ambulation (Consroe and Sandyk, 1992). "A new skeletal muscle relaxant would be most welcome" (Hollister, 1986).

Drugs for bladder dysfunction

Antimuscarinic drugs (e.g. oxybutynin, flavoxate, propantheline) are used to treat urinary frequency. They increase bladder capacity by decreasing detrusor muscle contractions. All may cause dry mouth, blurred vision, constipation, difficulty in micturition and may precipitate glaucoma.

Cholinergic agents (e.g. carbachol, bethanechol, distigmine) are used for bladder hypotonia. They improve voiding efficiency by increasing detrusor muscle contraction. Adverse effects, though less acute for distigmine, are due to generalised parasympathomimetic activity such as sweating, nausea, vomiting, blurred vision, bradycardia and intestinal colic. Combinations of antimuscarinics, alpha-adrenergic antagonists and/or muscle relaxants are sometimes helpful, but also have numerous side effects.

Bladder dysfunction is almost universal in long-standing MS and common in spinal cord injuries. The available drugs are not very effective and management is difficult. It would clearly be helpful to find a single drug that is effective both for muscle spasticity and bladder dysfunction.

Drugs for pain relief in spastic conditions

Acute pain syndromes are not uncommon in MS (see also Pain p.39-41 and Epilepsy p.49-53). These can be managed in most (though not all) cases with carbamazepine, alone or in combination with phenytoin or baclofen. Chronic pain, often occurring at night, is frequent in MS and spinal cord injuries and is more difficult to manage. It may fail to respond fully to carbamazepine, phenytoin, baclofen, tricyclic antidepressants, clonazepam, or nonsteroidal anti-inflammatory drugs, alone or in combination. Narcotic drugs, non-pharmacological treatments such as transcutaneous nerve stimulation and behavioural approaches may be required (Consroe and Sandyk, 1992).

There is a need for a drug which provides better analgesia, especially for central pain and especially at night, for these conditions.

Cannabis and cannabinoids in spastic disorders

Use in multiple sclerosis (MS) *(Table iii)*

Several anecdotal reports, including three described by Grinspoon and Bakalar (1993) and others in the press (Davies, 1992; Doyle, 1992; Ferriman, 1993; Handscombe, 1993; Hodges, 1992, 1993; James, 1993) suggest that cannabis can alleviate symptoms in patients with MS after other drugs have failed or produce unacceptable side effects (Appendix II).

A number of clinical studies have lent some weight to these reports although few patients have been studied and the results have not always been favourable. There have only been three double-blind, placebo-controlled studies involving more than one patient. Petro and Ellenberger (1981) studied nine patients with MS and found that 5-10mg THC given orally significantly reduced objectively rated spasticity compared with placebo (Fig. 4).

However, only three patients felt subjectively improved ("loose and better able to walk"); one of these had not improved by objective criteria. Ungerleider et al. (1988) observed 12 MS patients and noted significant subjective improvement compared with placebo at doses of 7.5mg of oral THC (Fig. 5), but no change in objective measurements of weakness, spasticity, coordination, gait or reflexes. Adverse effects were common and most of the patients did not request further treatment with THC. Greenberg et al. (1994) measured the effect of smoking cannabis on postural

Figure 4: Change in clinically rated spasticity score after THC in 9 patients with multiple sclerosis (Petro and Ellenberger, 1981)

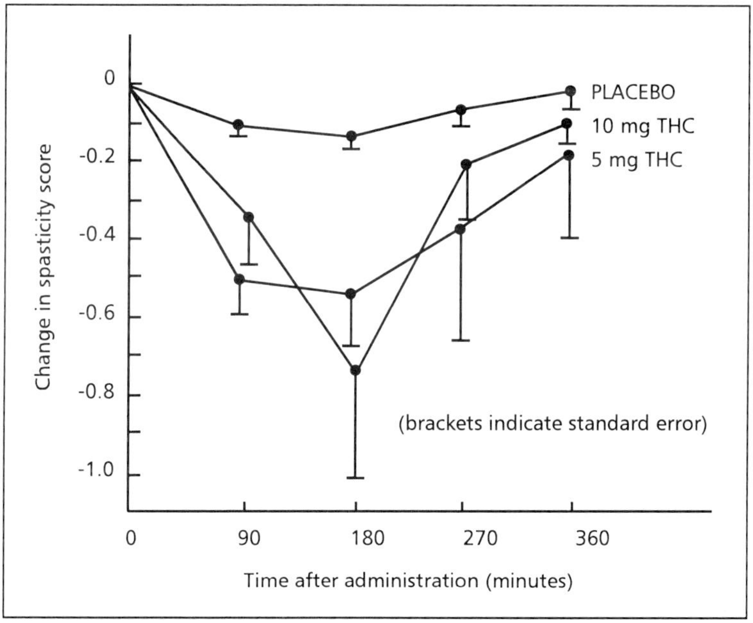

Figure 5: Individual subjective ratings of spasticity after different doses of THC in 12 patients with multiple sclerosis (Ungerleider et al., 1988). *The dotted and solid lines, and different styles of points are used to distinguish individual patients and are not otherwise significant*

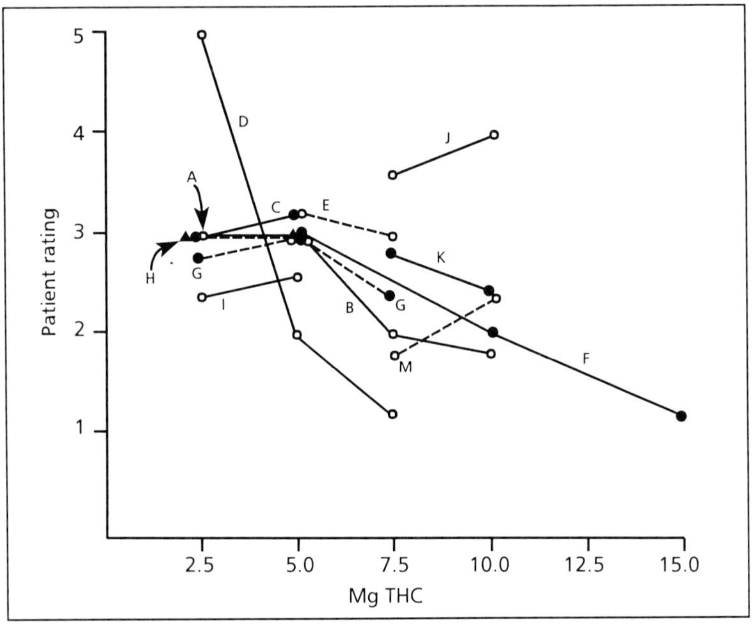

control in 10 patients with MS and 10 normal controls and found that cannabis impaired posture and balance in all subjects, the effect being greatest in the patients, who became further impaired. There were no other objective changes on neurological examination, but some patients noted subjective improvement.

Clifford (1983) conducted an open trial in eight patients with severe MS who received placebo or 5-15mg oral THC 6-hourly for up to 18 hours. Five patients showed mild subjective but not objective improvement in tremor and well-being on THC. Two patients showed both subjective and objective improvement in tremor but not in ataxia or other symptoms. There was a remarkable improvement in tremor and hand coordination in one of these (Fig. 6). All patients experienced a "high" and two became

Figure 6: Handwriting sample and movement artefact from head, recorded before and ninety minutes after ingestion of 5mg THC in patient with multiple sclerosis (Clifford, 1983)

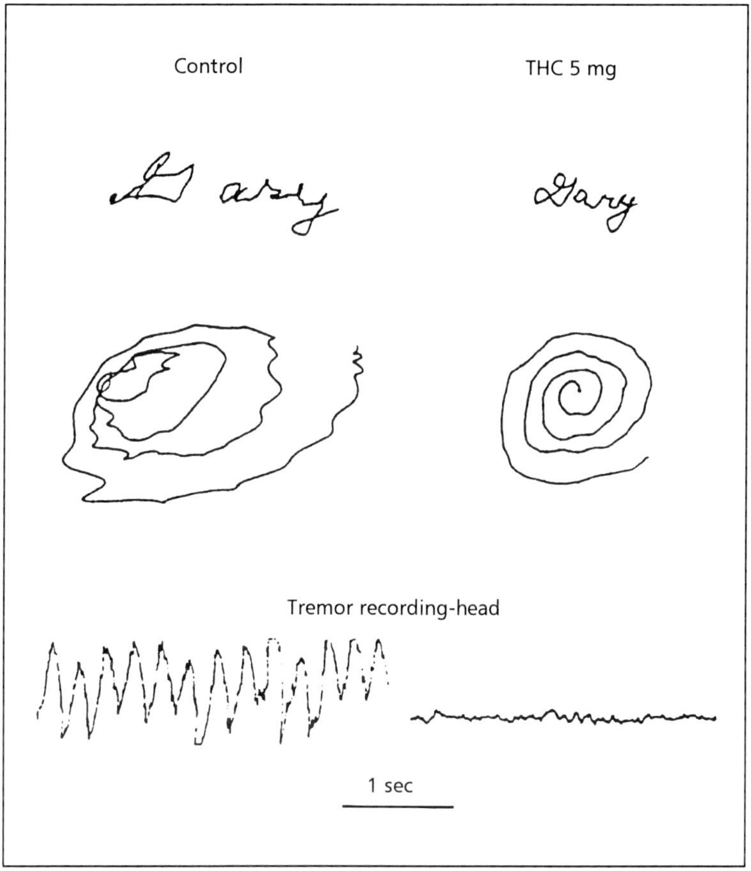

dysphoric. A single open case study was reported by Meinck et al. (1989). The patient's spasticity, ataxia and tremor (Fig. 7) improved after smoking a cannabis cigarette. Martyn et al. (1995) reported the effects of nabilone in a double-blind, placebo-controlled crossover study of one patient with MS. The patient took 1mg nabilone every second day for two periods of four weeks, alternating with four week periods of placebo. There was a clear

Figure 7: Electromagnetic recording of the finger and hand action tremor in a pointing task on the morning before and the evening after smoking a marihuana cigarette in a patient with multiple sclerosis (Meinck et al., 1989)

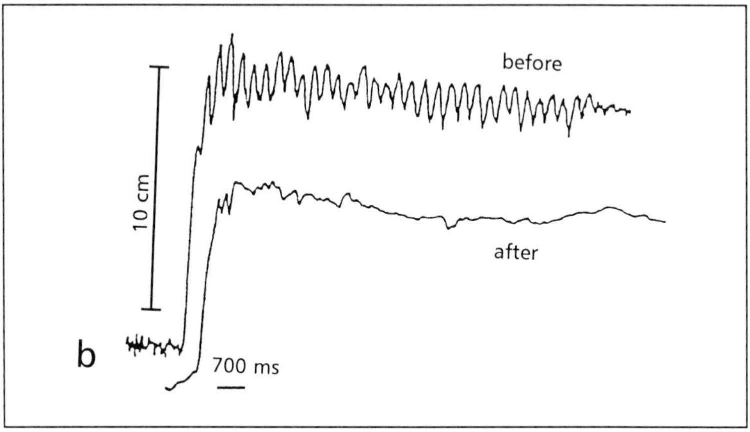

improvement in general well-being, muscle spasms and frequency of nocturia during the two periods on nabilone (Fig. 8).

Finally, a questionnaire study by Consroe et al. (1996) supported the impression given by anecdotal reports that a considerable number of MS patients take cannabis covertly for symptom relief. Questionnaires enquiring about cannabis use were sent to 233 MS patients in the UK and USA. The response rate was 48% (112 patients) and patients reported taking cannabis for spasticity, muscle pain and spasms especially at night, depression, anxiety, tremor, paraesthesia, numbness, weakness, impaired balance, constipation and memory loss.

Use in spinal cord injury *(Table iv)*

Patients with spinal cord injuries often have symptoms similar to those of MS including spasticity, painful muscle spasms, and impaired bladder control. A few papers report alleviation of symptoms in these patients with cannabis or THC. Dunn and

Figure 8: Symptoms while receiving nabilone or placebo in a patient with multiple sclerosis (Martyn et al., 1995)

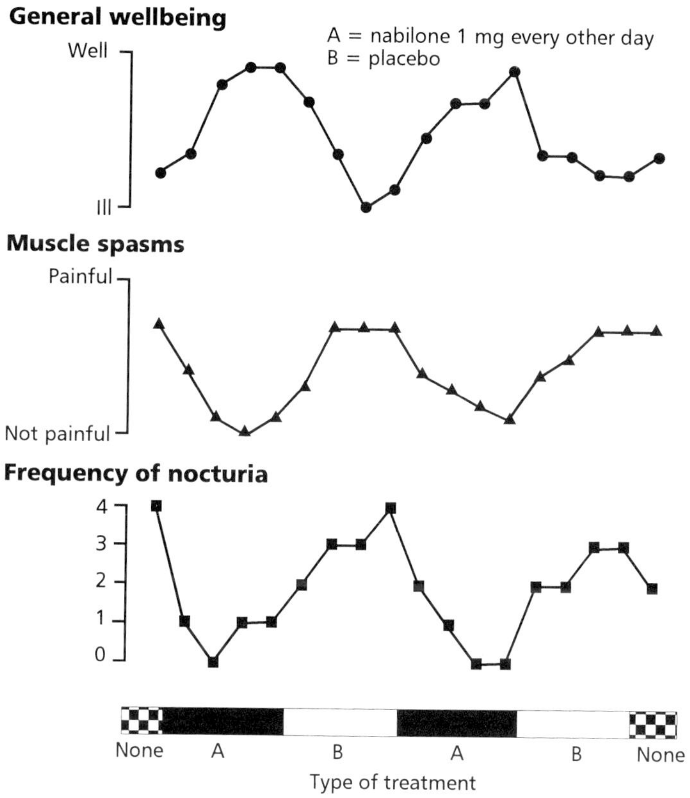

Davis (1974) surveyed the perceived effects of cannabis in 10 patients with a range of problems arising from spinal cord injury. The results were mixed: five out of eight with spasticity and five out of nine with headache noted improvement; four out of nine with phantom limb pain noted improvement but two out of ten reported worsening of urinary symptoms. Petro (1980) reported on a patient with spinal cord injury for whom cannabis relieved pain and muscle spasms. Malec et al. (1982) conducted a questionnaire survey which indicated that 21 of 24 patients with spinal cord injuries who had used cannabis found that it decreased spasticity. The only double-blind controlled trial (Maurer et al., 1990) concerned a single patient in whom oral THC (5mg) was compared with oral codeine (50mg) and placebo, each administered 18 times over five months. Codeine and THC alleviated pain to a similar degree and were better than placebo, but the THC had an additional beneficial effect on spasticity.

Use in movement disorders *(Table iv)*

Consroe and Snider, (1986) investigated the effect of cannabidiol (100-600mg/day over six weeks) in an open trial of five patients with various dystonias. There was a 20-50% improvement in dystonia in all cases, but tremor and hypokinesia was exacerbated in two patients with coexisting Parkinsonism. Sandyk and Awerbuch (1988) published case reports on three patients with Tourette's syndrome: the patients reported some relief of their tics when they smoked cannabis, but the authors suggested that this was due to anxiolytic rather than antidyskinetic effects of cannabis. Frankel et al. (1990) compared cannabis smoking with other drugs in five patients with Parkinson's disease and found that it produced no beneficial effects. Consroe et al. (1991) similarly found no beneficial effects of cannabidiol in 15 patients with Huntington's disease. Finally, cannabis has been advocated for extrapyramidal symptoms and tardive dyskinesia caused by phenothiazines in schizophrenic patients (Biezanek, 1994), although there have been no formal investigations.

Studies reviewed by Consroe and Sandyk (1992) suggest that cannabis misuse, which is common in schizophrenics (Negrete et al., 1986; Meuser et al., 1990), is not a risk factor for neuroleptic-induced tardive dyskinesia or Parkinsonism. However, in their review article, Cantwell and Harrison show that cannabis can have an adverse effect on the outcome of psychotic illness. Among schizophrenic patients misusing cannabis, such use is associated with a greater severity of psychotic symptoms, and earlier and more frequent relapses (Cantwell and Harrison, 1996).

Research needed

It is somewhat paradoxical that cannabinoids are reported to be of therapeutic value in neurological disorders associated with spasticity, ataxia, muscle weakness and tremor, since very similar symptoms can be caused by cannabis itself (Section 4 and Table 3). Frequent side-effects of acute doses of cannabis, THC, nabilone and other cannabinoids in normal subjects are ataxia, incoordination, tremulousness, muscle weakness and, at higher doses, myoclonic jerks (Consroe and Snider, 1986; Consroe and Sandyk, 1992). Slowing of reaction times and impaired psychomotor performance are almost universal (Hollister, 1986). Motor stretch reflexes are either increased or unchanged in man (Consroe and Snider, 1986), although cannabinoids attenuate certain reflexes and inhibit motor function in some animals (Pertwee, 1990).

However, it is not clear how much of the reputed effects of cannabis in motor disorders are due to psychoactive or analgesic effects, and a great deal of further research is needed to clarify their actions in such conditions. In view of the poor symptom control achieved by available drugs in many cases, such research is a matter of some urgency. It is ironic that the commonest neurological causes of taking illicit cannabis in the USA and UK are MS and spinal cord injury (Consroe and Sandyk, 1992; Beddow, 1995), yet only four controlled trials involving more than one patient have been published.

The required research should take the form of properly controlled trials on larger numbers of patients, with careful measurement of both subjective and objective changes. On present evidence it appears that cannabinoids could be helpful for particular symptoms in some patients (possibly as adjuvants to other drugs) but might aggravate symptoms in others. Trials of a range of cannabinoids including THC, nabilone, and possibly more selective synthetic cannabinoids (Consroe and Sandyk, 1992) may also be worth pursuing. Because the neurological disorders for which cannabis is reported to be of use are not of one primary origin, it is important that accurately described lesions are studied and strict recruitment criteria used in clinical trials.

A further problem with long-term use of cannabinoids in chronic diseases is the development of tolerance. Long-term trials with regular dosing are needed to investigate this question, and also to reveal any adverse effects of long-term cannabinoid use. Controlled trials to date have been limited to short-term studies, yet for chronic progressive diseases, such as MS, treatment for life (perhaps intermittently) may be required. The mode of administration is also important: smoking cannabis is clearly undesirable because of toxic constituents in the smoke (Table 2), while oral administration has the drawback of slow and irregular absorption (see Pharmacokinetics, p.11-15) Trials with different dosages and formulations of cannabinoids are needed to establish optimal regimens, which may need to be individualised.

Conclusions

- Cannabinoids may have a potential use for patients with spastic neurological disorders such as MS and spinal cord injury. Such patients often have distressing symptoms which are not well controlled with available drugs.
- Carefully controlled trials of cannabinoids in patients with chronic spastic disorders which have not responded to other drugs are indicated. Such trials merit a high priority.

- Depending on the results of such trials there may be a case for considering extension of the indications for nabilone (and allowing THC) for use on a named patient basis, in chronic spastic disorders unresponsive to standard drugs.
- Study groups should follow up their patients long term (i.e. years later) in order to evaluate adverse effects.

Pain

Pain is perhaps the commonest of all medical symptoms requiring drug treatment. Many analgesics, some ancient and time-honoured, others recently introduced, are available for the treatment of various types of pain. Although these are effective in most cases, there are still many patients in whom pain control is incomplete. Pain mechanisms are generated by both central nervous system activity and the peripheral nervous system. Nociceptive pain, much of which originates in the inflammatory reactions around sites of injury, but where the nervous system is intact, can be intractable but generally responds to drug therapy with anti-inflammatory drugs. However, drug therapy for nociceptive pain is often contraindicated, such as with nonsteroidal analgesia, or may have unwanted side effects, such as nausea and vomiting with opioids. Neuropathic pain, which results from damage to the nervous system, such as nerve invasion by cancer cells, is more often intractable and, by definition, more difficult to treat. However, clinically pain can have both nociceptive and neuropathic components, for instance in cancer patients. (Physical treatments for pain such as electrical stimulation techniques and acupuncture are not discussed here).

Existing pharmacological treatments

Non-opioid analgesics include aspirin, paracetamol, nefopam and anti-inflammatory analgesics such as ibuprofen and many others. These are suitable for a wide variety of mild to moderate pains. They are generally safe but all have certain drawbacks. Gastrointestinal irritation and bleeding may present a problem with aspirin and other non-steroidal anti-inflammatory agents and some patients are unable to take them because of hypersensitivity. Paracetamol can cause severe liver damage in overdose, which may occur with as few as 15-20 tablets taken at once. Nefopam may cause troublesome side-effects including nervousness, insomnia, dry mouth, sweating, blurred vision and others.

Opioid analgesics include codeine, dextropropoxyphene, morphine, diamorphine (heroin), methadone, pethidine, pentacozine, fentanyl and others. Codeine and dextropropoxyphene are suitable for mild or moderate pain; the others are all potent analgesics used for moderate or severe pain especially pain of visceral origin. All opioid analgesics commonly cause nausea, vomiting, constipation and drowsiness. Euphoria or dysphoric states also occur. Larger doses can produce respiratory depression and hypotension. Tolerance to the analgesic effects occurs and dosage needs to be adjusted if the drugs are used long-term for chronic pain. All these drugs can cause physical dependence and have potential misuse liability, although this is rarely a problem when they are used for analgesia.

Drugs for neuralgic pain Anticonvulsant drugs such as carbamazepine (see Epilepsy p.49-54) are sometimes effective for trigeminal neuralgia; tricyclic antidepressants (e.g. amitriptyline) may be effective in postherpetic neuralgia, oral and facial pains, some chronic pain syndromes and pain of central origin, often in combination with other drugs.

Drugs for migraine include aspirin and paracetamol, ergotamine and sumatriptan as well as various drug combinations and antiemetic drugs. Difficulties in absorption hamper the use of oral analgesics and ergotamine and the value of ergotamine is limited by side-effects including nausea, vomiting, abdominal pain and muscle cramps. Sumatriptan is effective but has a high rebound attack rate. It cannot be taken with ergotamine and may cause severe chest pain and tightness mimicking angina pectoris.

Drugs for terminal care Various combinations of drugs — opioids, neuroleptics (phenothiazines), laxatives, antidepressants, anti-inflammatory agents, and anticonvulsants — are used for chronic and acute pains in terminal care with the aim of alleviating pain while avoiding excessive drowsiness and constipation caused by opioids.

Despite recent advances, it would be complacent to believe that problems in pain control are solved. In fact, Segal (1986, p.106) claims that "the lack of adequate pain relief still heads the list of unresolved medical problems". New drugs with minimal toxicity and efficacy in types of pain not well controlled by standard drugs could strengthen the analgesic armamentarium, either singly or in combination with existing drugs.

Cannabis and cannabinoids as analgesics *(Table v)*

Many cannabinoids have analgesic and anti-inflammatory properties in animal models (reviewed by Segal, 1986 and Consroe and Sandyk, 1992). "Unfortunately the cannabinoid receptor appears to be coupled to both analgesic and cannabinimimetic activities, and, thus far, the bond seems to be largely inseparable" (Consroe and Sandyk, 1992, p. 468). Segal also found only psychoactive cannabinoids to have analgesic activity. However, this is contradicted by Evans' report that cannabidiol, also non-psychoactive, is a powerful analgesic but limited by a ceiling effect (Evans, 1991) (Table 1). Two synthetic compounds, still experimental, Δ^8-THC-11-oic acid and the synthetic cannabinoid (-)-HU-210, possibly separate analgesic and cannabinimimetic activities but have not been tested in man (Consroe and Sandyk, 1992) (Table 1).

The antinociceptive and anti-inflammatory effects of cannabinoids in animals have led to a few trials in various types of human pain. In addition, the anti-epileptic properties of cannabinoids (see Epilepsy, p.49-54) have suggested that they might be useful in some types of paroxysmal pain which respond better to anticonvulsant drugs such as carbamazepine than to non-steroidal anti-inflammatory agents or opiate analgesics.

Nevertheless, the number of human trials is limited and the results somewhat equivocal. Noyes et al. (1975a and b) carried out two double-blind placebo-controlled studies with oral THC. In the first study (1975a) 10 patients with cancer pain received doses of 5, 10, 15 and 20mg THC and placebo in random order. Significant pain relief was obtained with the two higher doses compared with placebo. Pain relief peaked at three hours and was still near maximum six hours after THC administration. Drowsiness and mental clouding were commonly observed with THC, but other psychoactive effects were described as minimal; euphoria was grossly evident in only two patients. In the second study (1975b) oral THC 10mg and 20mg was compared with oral codeine 60 and 120mg in 36 patients with cancer pain. Analgesic efficacy was equivalent with the two drugs and both THC 20mg and codeine 120mg gave significant pain relief compared with placebo. These results were supported by a single case double-blind, placebo-controlled study (Maurer, 1990) who found that oral THC 5mg and codeine 50mg gave similar pain relief in a patient with spinal cord injury. Jain et al. (1981) in another controlled study reported significant pain relief compared to placebo in 56 patients with postoperative pain given the synthetic cannabinoid levonantradol intramuscularly in four doses (1.5, 2, 2.5 and 3mg). There was no clear dose-response effect but analgesia with the higher doses persisted for well over six hours. Drowsiness was a common side-effect but there were few if any psychoactive effects. The prolonged duration of effect noted in some of these studies may be therapeutically useful when compared with available analgesics.

In contrast, Raft et al. (1977) found no significant analgesic effects from two doses of intravenous THC (0.22mg/kg and 0.44mg/kg in 10 healthy patients undergoing dental surgery (wisdom tooth extraction). In fact in these patients the higher dose of THC was rated as least effective in alleviating postoperative pain, and diazepam 0.157mg/kg as most effective. Six subjects preferred placebo to THC; four preferred low dose THC to placebo. A negative result was also reported by Lindstrom et al. (1987) in 10 patients with chronic neuropathic pain (causalgia, postherpetic neuralgia etc) given oral cannabidiol 450mg/day in divided doses.

Some types of pain may respond to cannabinoids better than others. Thus in a survey by Dunn and Davis (1974) four respondents reported improvement in phantom limb pain after taking cannabis and Finnegan-Ling and Musty (1994) described another case relieved by THC. Grinspoon and Bakalar (1993) give three anecdotal reports of the analgesic effects of cannabis in one patient with a brain tumour and two with rare painful conditions (Appendix II). In addition they describe alleviation of migraine by cannabis in one patient. Consroe and Sandyk (1992) give a theoretical reason for a possible therapeutic role for cannabinoids in migraine, since THC and cannabidiol inhibit serotonin release (thought to be a factor in migraine) *in vitro* from human platelets taken during a migrainous attack but not between attacks. However, there have been no studies of the effect of cannabinoids in migraine.

Research needed

THC has been shown in well controlled studies to have significant analgesic effects in patients with chronic pain due to cancer (Noyes et al., 1975 a,b), and the synthetic cannabinoid levonantradol appears to be effective in postoperative pain (Jain et al., 1981), although there was no clear dose-response relationship. Further research on these compounds for chronic and postoperative pain after major surgery seems justified, and other less psychoactive cannabinoids could profitably be investigated. However, experience with opiates has shown that psychoactive effects (e.g. euphoria or addiction) are not important considerations in treating patients with terminal (e.g. cancer pain) or short-lived (e.g. postoperative) pain conditions.

Cannabinoids may also prove useful as adjunctive drugs, used in combination with standard analgesics, in chronic painful conditions and in terminal care. An adjunctive role seems the most likely since the potency of THC alone appears to be approximately equivalent to that of codeine (Noyes et al., 1975b) which is only moderately potent as an analgesic. The analgesic action of cannabinoids appears to be mediated by a non-opioid mechanism (Segal, 1986; Lal et al., 1981).

Hospices and surgical wards would be ideal settings for carefully controlled studies of cannabinoids, in comparison with and in combination with other drugs for these indications. In addition, pain control clinics might provide a good testing ground for trials of cannabinoids for phantom limb pain, a condition notoriously difficult to treat with standard analgesics.

There is less evidence at present in favour of trials of cannabinoids in migraine or in conditions, such as rheumatic pain, where their anti-inflammatory effects might theoretically be useful. It seems clear that presently available cannabinoids are not useful in routine dental surgery (Raft et al., 1977). However, continued active research on novel synthetic cannabinoids with increased analgesic potency (Johnson and Melvin, 1986) should be encouraged.

Conclusions

- Some cannabinoids (THC and levonantradol) have undoubted analgesic effects.
- Further research on the use of cannabinoids in chronic and terminal pain, various neuropathic pains including phantom limb pain, and postoperative pain is justified. Hospices, pain control clinics and postoperative surgical wards could provide ideal settings for such research.
- It seems likely that cannabinoids (including new more selective synthetic agents such as levonantradol, (-)-HU-210 and others in the process of development) serve a useful role in pain control, especially as adjuncts to standard analgesics in pain conditions not well controlled by standard analgesic drugs.
- There may be a case for permitting the use of THC and nabilone for intractable pain, especially in terminal illness.

Anorexia (Loss of appetite) *(Table vi)*

Effects of cannabis and cannabinoids on appetite

Cannabis has been reported to increase appetite in man although the mechanism is unknown and the evidence mixed (Mattes et al., 1994). As reviewed by Paton and Pertwee (1973), acute doses in normal subjects are followed about three hours later by increased appetite, delayed satiation, and increased "relish" for food, especially sweet foods. With chronic administration or large doses, the stimulant effect on appetite disappears and depression of appetite ensues.

Trials on patients with anorexia from various causes have had mixed results. THC appears to be ineffective in anorexia nervosa. Gross et al., (1983) in a prospective, randomised, double-blind crossover trial found that there was no difference in weight gain between oral THC (7.5- 30mg daily) and diazepam (3-15mg daily), each administered for two weeks, in 11 patients with primary anorexia nervosa. THC caused severe dysphoric reactions in three of the patients.

Since anorexia nervosa does not appear to be characterised by a lack of appetite but by an overpowering compulsion to refuse food despite feeling hungry, it is unsurprising that THC is ineffective for this condition. One might speculate that dysphoric reactions in these patients may be because THC does, in fact, increase their appetite and thus intensifies their mental conflict between hunger and food refusal.

More positively, the anti-emetic effects of THC may allow eating and prevent weight loss in patients undergoing cancer chemotherapy (see Nausea and vomiting associated with cancer chemotherapy, p.21-23). There are some reports that THC can have similar effects in patients with AIDS-related diseases, many of whom are receiving antiviral drugs such as zidovudine, or have hepatitis, and other illnesses which cause anorexia, nausea and vomiting. Plasse et al. (1991) reported an open study on 10 patients with AIDS-related diseases, receiving antiviral therapy. The patients received dronabinol (THC in sesame oil) orally 2.5mg up to three times a day "as needed" for five months. Prior to treatment, the patients were losing a median of 0.93kg/month; on treatment they gained 0.54kg/month, a significant difference. In a follow-up study, Beal et al. (1995) compared dronabinol (2.5mg twice daily) with placebo in 72 patients with advanced AIDS-related illness. Dronabinol, but not placebo, significantly reduced nausea, increased appetite, prevented further weight loss and improved mood (Fig. 9a and b). As a result of this study,

Figure 9a: Mean change in appetite from baseline in patients with AIDS treated with dronabinol (THC) and placebo (Beal et al., 1995)

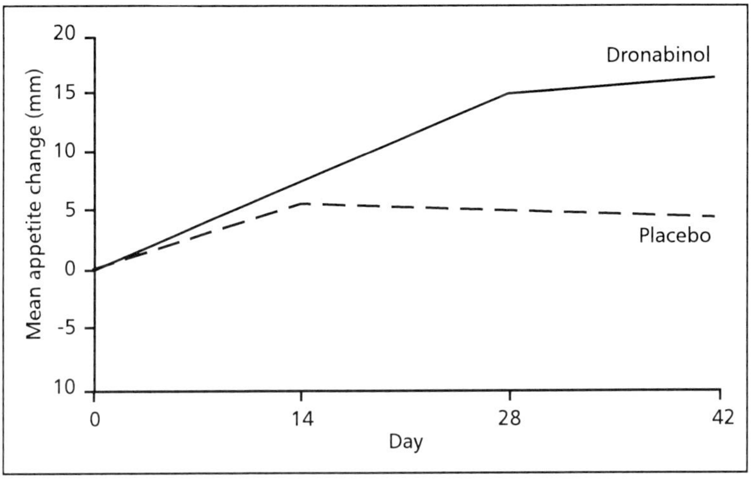

Figure 9b: Mean change in weight from baseline in patients with AIDS treated with dronabinol (THC) and placebo (Beal et al., 1995)

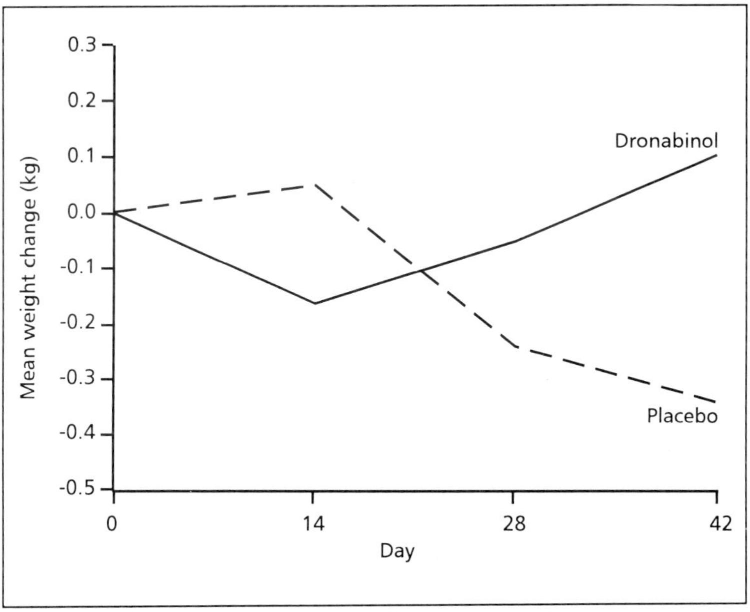

dronabinol was approved by the American Food and Drug Administration for use in anorexia associated with AIDS. Although anorexia with weight loss may occur with nausea and vomiting, they may not all respond to the same therapy. For instance nabilone, while effective as an anti-emetic, does not stimulate appetite.

In addition to these studies, anecdotal reports of benefits from smoked cannabis in AIDS patients, two of whom were unable to tolerate ziduvodine, are given by Grinspoon and Bakalar (1993) (Appendix II).

Research needed

It is not clear whether the apparent stimulation of appetite by cannabinoids is separate from the anti-emetic effect, but further trials of THC, nabilone, other cannabinoids, and combinations of cannabinoids with other anti-emetics such as prochlorperazine in conditions such as AIDS and cachexia due to malignant disease are warranted.

A concern with regard to the use of cannabinoids in AIDS and cancer chemotherapy patients is that cannabinoids have been shown to have immunosuppressive effects (see Effects of chronic dosage with cannabinoids relevant to therapeutic use, p.67-70). Such effects may be potentially damaging in individuals whose immune system is already compromised by HIV or chemotherapy, especially if used long term. A prospective study failed to find any relationship between cannabis use and the rate of development of clinical AIDS in HIV-positive men (Kaslow et al., 1989). Nevertheless, as pointed out by Hall et al. (1994), the issue of immunosuppression needs to be explicitly investigated in any research on the use of cannabinoids in the treatment of AIDS, and cancer.

Conclusions

- THC appears to be helpful in preventing weight loss in AIDS-related diseases.
- Allowing the prescription of nabilone and THC for cancer chemotherapy and HIV/AIDS seems justified for preventing weight loss and treating anorexia in HIV/AIDS irrespective of whether the patient is experiencing nausea and/or vomiting.

Epilepsy

Epilepsy affects about 1% of the population, and about 200,000 people in the UK are taking antiepileptic drugs. However, the drugs provide total protection from convulsions in only about two-thirds of patients; in about a third control is unsatisfactory and some of these patients are severely and permanently disabled. In addition, the drugs must usually be taken long-term, sometimes for life, and all can produce adverse effects which can be severe.

Existing pharmacological treatments

First-line drugs

Sodium valproate. Effective for generalised and partial seizures. Unwanted effects include weight gain, hair thinning, and tremor; rarely hepatotoxicity, thrombocytopenia and pancreatitis occur.

Carbamazepine. Effective for generalised and partial seizures. Unwanted effects include dizziness, nausea and other gastrointestinal disturbances, headache, visual disturbances and drowsiness. Skin rash develops in some patients. Severe but rare idiosyncratic reactions include Stevens-Johnson syndrome, toxic epidermal necrolysis and hepatitis.

Second-line drugs

Phenytoin. Effective for generalised and partial seizures. Adverse effects are common and include insomnia, mental confusion, and headache; also ataxia, acne, hirsutism, facial coarsening and rarely haematological effects. Dosage is difficult to control.

Phenobarbitone, primidone. Effective for all types of seizures but regularly cause central nervous system depression and are reserved for patients who cannot tolerate other drugs.

Add-on drugs

Vigabatrin, lamotogrine, gabapentin and topiramate. Have been introduced relatively recently and are usually used as adjunctive therapy for partial or generalised seizures (although vigabatrin and lamotogrine have been licensed for monotherapy in certain conditions). Vigabatrin can cause drowsiness, fatigue, irritability, weight gain and psychosis which limit its use. Lamotrigine can cause skin rashes in some patients, and rarely a severe allergic rash. Gabapentin can cause somnolence, dizziness and ataxia, and topiramate can cause ataxia, impaired concentration and confusion.

Clobazam, clonazepam. These are benzodiazepines and are best used intermittently since tolerance develops with continued use; sedation is common and withdrawal seizures may be a problem.

Ethosuximide. Useful in childhood absence and atypical seizures; no action on generalised tonic-clonic or partial seizures. Side-effects include gastrointestinal disturbances, drowsiness, dizziness, headache, depression and mild euphoria. Rarely psychotic states, blood disorders, hepatic and renal changes and other adverse effects occur.

The treatment of epilepsy has greatly improved in recent years with the introduction of new drugs such as lamotogrine and gabapentin, and new drugs are still being developed. However, adverse effects are common and interactions between different antiepileptic drugs can be a problem, especially with add-on therapies. First and second line drugs, and benzodiazepines, can have adverse effects on the foetus if taken by the mother during pregnancy. Furthermore, there remains a sizable core of patients, 20-30%, in whom seizure control is incomplete. There is a need for an efficient anticonvulsant drug which is relatively free of adverse effects, especially generalised central nervous system depression.

Cannabis and cannabinoids in epilepsy *(Table vii)*

Animal work, reviewed by Consroe and Snider (1986) and Consroe and Sandyk (1992), shows that cannabinoids have complex actions on seizure activity, and that they can exert both anticonvulsant and proconvulsant effects. In particular, cannabidiol has been suggested to be a promising candidate as an antiepileptic drug since it appears to have a spectrum of anticonvulsant properties different from THC and from standard drugs and to have few psychoactive effects (Hollister, 1986). However, information on the possible therapeutic effects of cannabinoids in human epilepsy is almost non-existent. There have been only a few reports over the past 150 years, and most are brief uncontrolled observations or studies in one or only a few patients (Consroe and Sandyk, 1992), with contradictory results.

Cannabis smoking appeared to precipitate convulsions in one epileptic patient who had been fit-free for six months without medication, although the causal relationship was not clear (Keeler and Reifler, 1967). However, in another single case report (Consroe et al, 1975) and two anecdotal reports (Grinspoon and

Bakalar, 1993) smoking cannabis appeared to alleviate seizures in patients with generalised, partial or absence seizures. Two of these subjects continued taking standard medication and one was able to reduce his dosage (Appendix II).

The only controlled trials have been carried out with cannabidiol. Cunha et al. (1980) found that 200-300mg/day of cannabidiol added to standard anticonvulsant therapy for four to five months improved seizure control in seven of eight patients with generalised epilepsy secondary to a temporal lobe focus. In contrast, Ames and Cridland (1986) and Trembly et al. (1990) found that this dosage of cannabidiol had no effect on seizure pattern or frequency over four weeks-six months. In one patient given cannabidiol 900-1200mg/day for 10 months in an open trial, Trembly et al. (1990) reported a reduction of seizure frequency.

Research needed

With such scanty human data , the role of cannabinoids as possible therapeutic agents in epilepsy remains speculative. It is unlikely that psychoactive cannabinoids such as THC, which have dual convulsant-anticonvulsant effects, will be therapeutically useful (Nahas, 1984). However, cannabidiol, which may act through a different mechanism since it does not interact with cannabinoid receptors (Pertwee, 1990) and has a different profile of anticonvulsant activity in animal models (Consroe and Snider, 1986), may have a therapeutic potential. It has the advantage of low psychoactivity, although it may produce sleepiness (Hall et al., 1994). It appears to have little anticonvulsant activity in man at doses of 200-300mg/day, but rigorous long-term well controlled trials with higher doses (900-1200mg/day) may be worth pursuing (Consroe and Sandyk, 1992). The present sparse evidence suggests that it could at least be a useful adjunctive treatment for patients not well controlled on standard anticonvulsant drugs. The available evidence suggests that tolerance does not occur with repeated use, but this possibility needs further investigation.

Conclusions

- Present pharmacotherapy for epilepsy is not fully satisfactory; better drugs with fewer adverse effects are needed.
- Evidence of a therapeutic potential for cannabinoids in epilepsy is scanty. Most trials have been small, uncontrolled, confused by use of other medications, and have given conflicting results.
- There is a theoretical potential for cannabidiol which may have anticonvulsant effects with minimal side-effects in large doses, and could possibly provide a useful adjunctive therapy for patients poorly controlled on presently available drugs. THC and other psychoactive cannabinoids are probably not suitable as anticonvulsants.

Glaucoma

Glaucoma is the commonest cause of blindness in the Western World. It is not a single disease but can result from many causes. The mechanisms involved are incompletely understood but may include vascular and neurodegenerative factors as well as raised intraocular pressure (IOP). The commonest form of glaucoma, primary open-angle glaucoma (chronic simple glaucoma), is characterised by a gradual increase in IOP possibly resulting from obstruction to the outflow of aqueous humour (Adler and Geller, 1986). Blindness ensues if the condition is untreated, but treatment is not always satisfactory.

Existing pharmacological treatments

Eye drops

Miotics are parasympathomimetic agents (e.g. pilocarpine, physostigmine, carbachol) which lower IOP by increasing the outflow of aqueous humour. Adverse effects include blurring of vision, headache, sweating, bradycardia, intestinal colic, hypersalivation and bronchospasm.

Adrenergic agents (e.g. adrenaline, dipivefrine, guanethidine) increase aqueous humour outflow and produce a modest decrease of IOP. Adverse effects include local irritation and conjunctival fibrosis.

Beta-blockers (e.g. timolol) lower IOP by decreasing the rate of aqueous humour formation. Adverse effects include local reactions in the eye; systemic effects contraindicate use in patients with asthma, bradycardia, heart block or heart failure.

Orally administered agents

Carbonic anhydrase inhibitors (e.g. acetazolamide, dichlorphenamide) decrease the formation of aqueous humour. Adverse effects include hypokalaemia, paraesthesia, lack of appetite, drowsiness and depression.

Most of these drugs are efficacious and the incidence of serious adverse effects is moderately low. However, none are ideal since tolerance develops to most of them. There is a need for improved pharmacotherapy for glaucoma, but it may not be possible to make rational advances until the mechanisms producing glaucoma are better understood.

Effects of cannabis and cannabinoids on intraocular pressure *(Table viii)*

Hepler and Frank (1971) reported that cannabis smoking lowered IOP in cannabis users. This observation was followed by several studies which showed that both smoked and orally administered cannabis (Hepler et al. 1976) and intravenous infusions of THC and various other cannabinoids (Perez-Reyes et al., 1976; Cooler and Gregg, 1977) could reduce IOP in normal subjects. Of the cannabinoids, only those with significant psychoactive and cardiovascular actions (Δ^8-THC, Δ^9-THC and 11-OH-THC) were effective; cannabinol, cannabidiol and beta-OH-THC produced only minimal reductions in IOP (Perez-Reyes et al., 1976). The results in humans were confirmed in numerous animal experiments, reviewed by Adler and Geller (1986).

Information on whether cannabinoids have a therapeutic potential in lowering intraocular pressure in patients with glaucoma is extremely sparse. Only two anecdotal reports and three small acute dosage studies on a total of 37 patients with glaucoma appear to have been published. There are no long-term studies. Grinspoon and Bakalar (1993) give anecdotal reports of two cases which received some notoriety in the US in the 1970s (Appendix II). Both individuals had glaucoma, although the type is not stated, and both obtained symptomatic relief and lowering of IOP, after standard pharmacotherapy had failed, from smoked or orally ingested cannabis in unspecified doses. Hepler et al. (1976) conducted a pilot open trial on 11 patients with glaucoma who smoked or took oral THC. Seven patients responded with a significant drop in IOP; THC had no effect in the other four. Only two double-blind controlled trials of THC in patients with glaucoma have been reported. Merritt et al. (1980) studied 18 patients administered with 2% THC by smoking. He observed a significant reduction in IOP (Fig. 10) but also noted hypotension, palpitations and psychotropic effects. These effects occurred with such frequency as to militate against the routine use of cannabis in

Figure 10: Intraocular pressure (IOP); mean ± standard error in 31 glaucoma eyes after cannabis and placebo inhalations (Merritt et al., 1980)

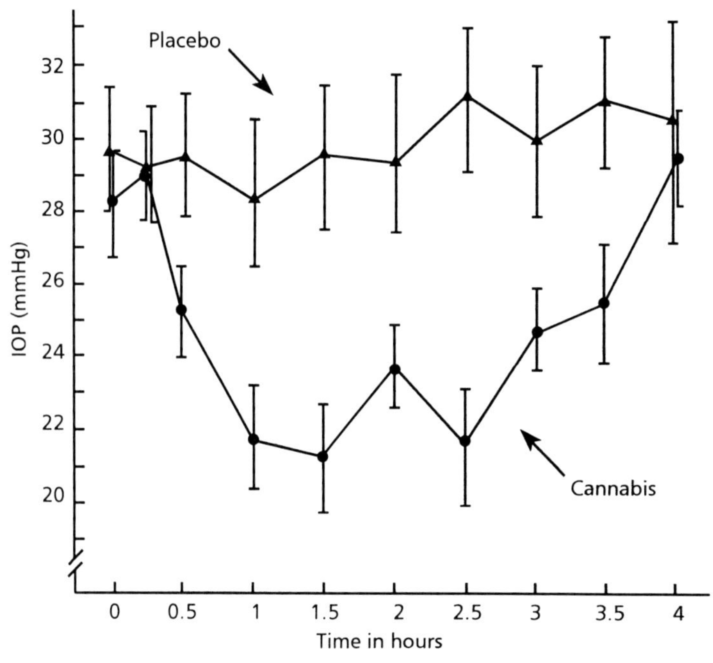

glaucoma. In a later small study of eight patients with glaucoma and vascular hypertension THC was administered to one eye in eye drops in concentrations of 0.01% (two patients), 0.05% and 0.1% (three patients each). The two stronger concentrations decreased IOP but the effect was observed in both eyes, suggesting a systemic mechanism of action despite the topical application. Mild hypotension but no psychoactive effects were observed.

Disadvantages of cannabinoids as treatment for glaucoma

Although these small studies suggest that cannabinoids can lower IOP in glaucoma, the mechanism of action is not known and there are several disadvantages of such a use. First, Jones et al. (1976; 1981) showed that tolerance develops to the effects of cannabis on IOP in normal subjects. Tolerance was apparent within 10 days of repeated oral administration of 10-30mg doses of THC, and there was a rebound in IOP to above baseline levels on cessation of dosage. Secondly, although topical application is the preferred mode of administration of drugs for glaucoma (to avoid generalised effects), it is difficult to prepare suitable solutions of cannabinoids since they are extremely lipid soluble/water insoluble. Green and Roth (1982) and Jay and Green (1983) found that topical administration of 1% THC in mineral oil produced no significant change in IOP in normal subjects.

Water-soluble compounds which exclude cannabinoids and have been identified as glycoproteins have been extracted from raw cannabis plant material and may provide hope of a new class of compounds being identified that are more active in reducing IOP than the cannabinoids (Green, 1982). A systemic effect from these compounds has been reported in an animal study through intravenous administration but no response to topical application (Green, 1982). Although Merritt et al. (1981) achieved an effect from local application it appeared that this was due to absorption into the general circulation. Indeed, the available evidence indicates that the effect of cannabinoids on IOP in man is due to systemic effects (Adler and Geller, 1986). (Effects obtained from local instillation into the eye in animals are probably not applicable to man because of interspecies differences in ocular dynamics). Unfortunately, all the cannabinoids which have been shown to lower IOP in men have undesirable psychoactive and cardiovascular effects.

In addition, cannabinoids have been reported to cause other ocular effects in man including photophobia, conjunctival hyperaemia, decreased lacrimation, corneal ulceration, conjunctivitis, keratitis and changes in pupil size (Adler and Geller, 1986). Since the effect of cannabinoids on IOP lasts five to six hours, they would need to be administered about four times daily, and Adler and Geller (1986) point out that, if used for the treatment of glaucoma, careful monitoring of the patient would be required for ocular effects as well as for systemic effects such as tachycardia, postural hypotension and central nervous system actions.

Research needed

Although the place of cannabinoids as treatment for glaucoma is doubtful at present, there are some areas where research might be fruitful. First, there appear to have been no trials comparing the beneficial/adverse effects of cannabinoids (such as THC, Δ^8-THC and nabilone) against those of existing agents. Larger carefully conducted studies are needed to establish the relative efficacy of cannabinoids in lowering IOP and the relative incidence of adverse effects compared to presently available drugs. Such studies would need to be fairly long-term to allow for the possible development of tolerance, which seems to occur with all existing drugs.

Secondly, there is some evidence that a variety of synthetic and semisynthetic cannabinoids may be able to lower IOP without side effects. These include Naboctate, a cannabinoid derivative (Razdan et al., 1983), and an orally effective analogue of THC which have both been tested in man, and several others which have shown promise in preclinical studies (Adler and Geller, 1986). Further basic research on these compounds, initially using suitable animal models, seems justified, since "there is the potential for dissociating the antiglaucoma from the CNS effects" of cannabinoids (Adler and Geller, 1986, p.62). It is also possible that cannabinoids have additive effects with other antiglaucoma agents and might have some use as adjunctive agents (Hollister, 1986).

Conclusions

- Present pharmacotherapy for glaucoma is not fully satisfactory; better drugs which cause fewer side-effects and less tolerance are needed.
- There seems little doubt that cannabinoids can reduce intraocular pressure in normal subjects, but claims for its therapeutic efficacy in patients with glaucoma rest on inadequate evidence. Only 26 patients with glaucoma have been studied in properly controlled trials; no comparisons have been made between cannabinoids and existing drugs, and no long-term trials have been conducted.
- There is a theoretical potential for certain cannabinoids to have a therapeutic use in glaucoma, but much further basic and clinical research in patients with glaucoma is needed to develop and investigate cannabinoids which lower intraocular pressure, preferably by topical application, without producing unacceptable systemic and CNS effects.

Bronchial Asthma *(Table ix)*

Existing pharmacological treatments

There is a national and international consensus about the prevention and management of asthma (British Thoracic Society et al, 1997; National Institute of Health, 1995) and such management, if properly instituted, is generally effective.

Pharmacological treatments include the use of bronchodilators (salbutamol, terbutaline, ipatropium, theophylline and others) and prophylactic measures including corticosteroids and sodium cromoglycate. Such drugs, though not devoid of side-effects, provide good control if used in suitable, stepwise combinations (British National Formulary, 1996). Emphasis is placed on prophylactic treatment to prevent the occurrence of severe asthmatic attacks. However, problems sometimes arise in steroid resistant cases, and acute severe asthma can be fatal if not treated promptly.

Cannabis and cannabinoids in asthma

Acute doses of cannabis and THC exert a definite bronchodilator effect on the small airways of the lungs (Hollister, 1986). The mechanism of this effect is not known but it appears to be different from that of the beta-adrenoceptor stimulants (e.g. salbutamol, terbutaline) and other drugs used at present as bronchodilators for asthma (Graham, 1986). Recent concern about risks associated with chronic use of beta-adrenoceptor stimulants has renewed interest in the possible use of cannabinoids for bronchial asthma.

However, there have been very few studies on the bronchodilator effects of cannabinoids in asthmatic patients. All of these were acute dose studies carried out in the 1970s. Tashkin et al. (1976) studied 14 asthmatic volunteers and compared smoked cannabis (2% THC), oral THC (15mg) and a standard bronchodilator isoprenaline (0.5%). They found that smoked cannabis and oral THC produced significant bronchodilatation of at least two hours duration. The effect of smoked cannabis was nearly equivalent to the clinical dose of isoprenaline. Smoked cannabis was also capable of reversing experimentally induced bronchospasm in three asthmatic subjects. However, smoking cannabis is clearly not a therapeutic option because of the smoke constituents other than THC it contains (Table 2), and oral THC is not considered suitable as a bronchodilator because of variations in the rate and extent of absorption. Furthermore, in effective doses it is apt to cause psychological disturbance (Graham, 1986).

Vachon et al. (1976) found that smoked THC (0.9% and 1.9%) produced significant and prolonged bronchodilatation in 17 asthmatic subjects, but the higher doses caused tachycardia. Williams et al. (1976) compared a THC aerosol containing 200 µg THC with a salbutamol aerosol (100 µg) in 10 asthmatic subjects. Both drugs significantly improved respiratory function. The onset of effect was more rapid with salbutamol, but the effects of both drugs were equivalent at one hour (Fig. 11). Tashkin et al. (1977) compared several doses of THC aerosol (5-20mg) with a standard

Figure 11: Comparison of the bronchodilator effect (increased FEV_1) of 100µg Salbutamol (•) and 200µg THC (o) inhaled as a metered dose aerosol in ten asthmatic subjects, double-blind with placebo (Williams et al., 1976)

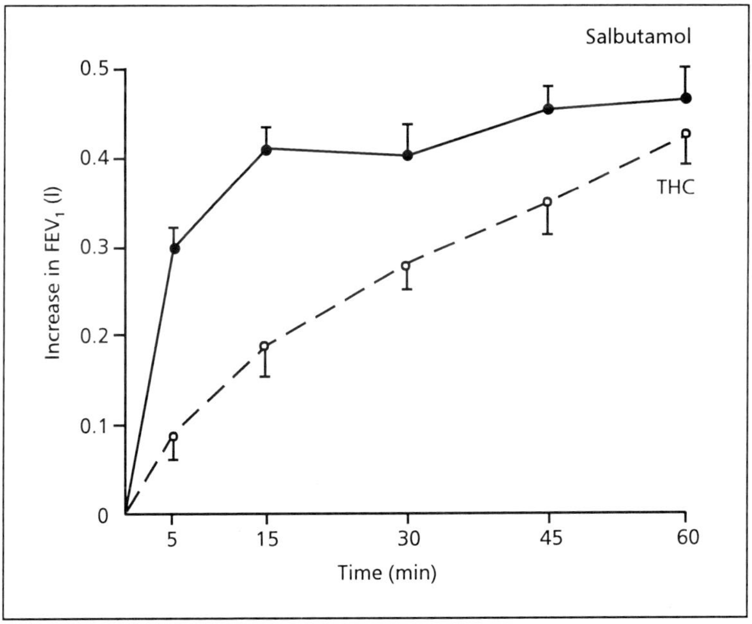

dose of isoprenaline in 11 normal volunteers and five asthmatic subjects. In the normal subjects and three of the asthmatics, the bronchodilator effect of THC was less than that of isoprenaline after five minutes. but significantly greater after one to three. However, in two of the asthmatics, the THC caused moderate to severe bronchoconstriction with coughing and chest discomfort. Three of the normal volunteers developed slight chest discomfort and cough. The authors concluded that the irritating effect of THC on the airways may make it unsuitable for therapeutic use.

Studies of the bronchodilator effect of other cannabinoids administered orally to normal volunteers (reviewed by Graham, 1986; Archer et al., 1986), have shown that Δ^8-THC has a bronchodilator effect comparable to THC with little cardiovascular or psychological effects; that cannabinol, cannabidiol and nabilone are ineffective, and that cannabidiol reduces the cardiovascular and psychological effects of THC without affecting the bronchodilator action.

Research needed

It seems clear that THC has bronchodilator actions and some scant evidence suggests that it can reverse airways constriction in some asthmatic subjects. However in other asthmatic patients THC may aggravate bronchospasm and cause coughing and chest discomfort. Present data is extremely limited and confined to acute dose studies in only a few asthmatic patients. Further studies would be required to confirm and extend the positive findings. In particular, a suitable form of administration needs to be developed. Graham (1986) suggests that a metered dose inhaler delivering 50-200μg THC may be effective, but it is not clear whether this dose will have irritant effects on the bronchial mucosa. Such a dose, locally administered, is unlikely to exert psychoactive effects.

Secondly, longer-term studies would be needed to see if tolerance develops in asthmatic subjects. Thirdly, the effects of combinations of cannabinoids with standard bronchodilators would have to be tested. Since cannabinoids appear to have a different mode of action from standard drugs, they could potentially be valuable for patients in whom the standard drugs provide inadequate control or cause excessive side-effects. Finally, there may be a potential for developing synthetic cannabinoids with selective bronchodilator effects without psychological or cardiovascular effects. However, such research does not appear to have a high priority; the main need for asthma at present is to develop better prophylactic treatments.

Conclusions

- Cannabinoids possibly have a potential as bronchodilators for patients with asthma, particularly as adjuvants to standard drugs.
- Further long-term studies using metered dose THC (or other synthetic cannabinoid) inhalers may be justified for patients unresponsive to existing drugs, but present evidence regarding efficacy is extremely limited.

Mood disorders, psychiatric conditions

Cannabis and cannabinoids have been advocated as antidepressants, anxiolytics, sedative/hypnotics, and as treatment for alcohol and opiate withdrawal syndromes. A few controlled studies have shown anxiolytic effects with nabilone (Fabre and McLendon, 1981; Ilaria et al., 1981), hypnotic effects with cannabidiol (Carlini and Cunha, 1981), and an antidepressant effect in cancer patients with THC (Regelson et al., 1976).

However, there is no convincing evidence of the general usefulness of cannabinoids, or their superiority over existing drugs, for these conditions. Animal work and some anecdotal reports suggest that THC and cannabinol can inhibit many of the signs of opioid withdrawal, by a non-opioid mechanism (Chesher and Jackson, 1985). This possibility may be worth pursuing in clinical studies to assist patients detoxifying from opiates.

Hypertension

The observation that cannabinoids cause postural hypotension (usually an unwanted effect) suggests a possible use as an antihypertensive agent. However, tolerance to the cardiovascular effects of cannabinoids (including those on blood pressure) develops rapidly and since they would have to be used long term, cannabinoids are unlikely to have a therapeutic use for hypertension (Jones et al., 1976; Benewitz and Jones, 1981).

4

Adverse effects of cannabis and cannabinoids in clinical use

The acute toxicity of cannabinoids is extremely low: they are very safe drugs and no deaths have been directly attributed to their recreational or therapeutic use. However, cannabinoids have actions on many body systems (Table 3) and, like all drugs, cause unwanted effects. Although some of these are frequent in medicinal use, they are not usually severe, and in this respect cannabinoids compare favourably with several other drugs (e.g. phenothiazines and other dopamine receptor antagonists, opioid and non-opioid analgesics, anticonvulsants) used for conditions in which cannabinoids have a potential therapeutic role. Centrally acting cannabinoids such as Δ^9-THC and nabilone generate the majority of unwanted effects; adverse effects relevant to the therapeutic uses of cannabinoids are summarised below.

Acute effects commonly observed in clinical settings

Sedation - drowsiness, dizziness, lethargy (incidence 50-100%). However, it is not known whether this only occurs in early doses or persists with continued dosage.

Psychological effects - euphoria ("high"), dysphoria, anxiety, feeling of loss of control, mental clouding, impaired memory (incidence 50-75%); depersonalisation, fear of dying, paranoia, hallucinations, depression, altered time-perception (less common but may be severe).

Physical symptoms and signs - dry mouth, ataxia (poor balance) (incidence over 50%); blurred vision, incoordination, muscle weakness, tremor, slurred speech, palpitations, tachycardia, hypotension, muscle twitching (less common); bronchospasm, chest discomfort, coughing (THC aerosols in asthma).

Other acute effects of cannabis relevant to therapeutic use

Impairment of psychomotor and cognitive performance, especially in complex tasks, has been shown in normal subjects in many tests (Paton and Pertwee, 1973; Nahas, 1984). Impairments include slowed reaction time, short term memory deficits, impaired attention, time and space distortion, impaired coordination. These effects combine with the sedative effects to cause deleterious effects on driving ability or operation of machinery. Because of the slow elimination of cannabinoids (see Pharmacokinetics, p.11-15) these effects may last for more than 24 hours after a single dose.

Interactions with other drugs. Additive effects are known to occur with other depressants including alcohol, benzodiazepines, opiates (Nahas, 1984), but further research is needed on drug interactions involving cannabinoids. This is particularly important for patients with complex diseases such as HIV/AIDS who may be taking several different drugs. Interactions may result not only from drugs with similar effects, but from competition for metabolic enzyme pathways.

Aggravation of psychosis in patients with schizophrenia with loss of control by antipsychotic drugs; possible precipitation of schizophrenia in vulnerable patients.

Effects of chronic dosage with cannabinoids relevant to therapeutic use

Tolerance has been shown to develop to many effects of cannabis in normal subjects. These include effects on mood, heart rate, blood pressure, salivary flow, intraocular pressure, EEG changes and psychomotor performance (Jones et al., 1976) and anti-emetic effects. Such tolerance can develop within weeks with repeated dosage though not at the same rate or degree for different effects (Pertwee, 1991). Tolerance can be an advantage in decreasing unwanted effects (e.g. dry mouth, dysphoria) but a disadvantage if a desired effect (e.g. anticonvulsant, decreased intraocular pressure) is involved. Further research is needed to determine whether tolerance can be overcome by raising the dose.

Dependence, withdrawal effects. Dependence is unlikely to present a problem with clinically prescribed doses for ill patients in therapeutic settings, but withdrawal effects may be undesirable. As well as psychological effects (restlessness, anxiety, insomnia, tremor), there may be a rebound rise in intraocular pressure, nausea, diarrhoea and other physical symptoms (Jones et al., 1976). Withdrawal symptoms are said to be short-lived (a few days) and mild in normal experimental subjects although they may be more severe in recreational users (Stephens et al., 1993). Withdrawal symptoms have not been studied in patients who use cannabis chronically for their therapeutic effects.

Whether the recreational use of cannabis encourages escalation of dosage and progression to other dependence-producing drugs remains debatable (Hall et al., 1994). However, experience with patients receiving opioids for pain relief shows that therapeutic use rarely leads to misuse (Twycross and McQuay, 1989) and the same is likely to be true of cannabis.

Endocrine effects. Cannabis and cannabinoids have complex effects on both male and female sex hormones and may present risks to the foetus if taken in pregnancy and exacerbate risk factors in labour (Hollister, 1986; Nahas, 1984).

Immunosuppressant effects. Animal studies suggest that cannabinoids interfere with various aspects of the immune system (Maykut, 1985). The significance of any such effects in man is not clear, but could be of importance in long-term use of cannabinoids in immunologically compromised patients. The existence of naturally occurring contaminants such as fungi and microbes in cannabis plants should also be considered.

Particular hazards of smoked cannabis. The smoke from herbal cannabis contains all the toxic constituents of cigarette smoke (apart from nicotine) including irritants, tumour initiators, tumour promotors and carcinogens, and carbon monoxide. The tar from cannabis smoke also contains greater concentrations of benzanthracenes and benzpyrenes (both carcinogens) than tobacco smoke (Table 2). It has been estimated that smoking a cannabis cigarette (containing only herbal cannabis) results in an approximately five-fold greater increase in carboxyhaemoglobin concentration, a three-fold greater increase in the amount of tar inhaled, and a retention in the respiratory tract of one third more tar than smoking a tobacco cigarette (Benson and Bentley, 1995). Thus chronic cannabis smoking, like tobacco smoking, increases the risk of cardiovascular disease, bronchitis, emphysema and probably carcinomas of the lung and aerodigestive tract (see Hall et al., 1995 for a review).

Cannabis versus cannabinoids. As mentioned in Section 2 (see constituents of cannabis, p.7-11) cannabis contains over 400 chemical compounds including more than 60 cannabinoids. Furthermore, there is considerable variation in the concentration of cannabinoids present in different preparations (Gough, 1991). Even if cannabis (either smoked or taken orally) from standardised preparations were shown to have therapeutic benefits, it would not be possible to know which particular agents (or combination of agents) were beneficial, and medical knowledge would not be advanced nor treatment improved. For these reasons, as well as the known toxic constituents in cannabis smoke mentioned above, it is considered here that cannabis is unsuitable for medical use. Such use should be confined to known dosages of pure or synthetic cannabinoids, given singly or sometimes in combination (e.g. THC and cannabidiol).

In addition to the many chemical compounds which make up the cannabis plant, street and illicit cannabis can contain both adulterants added by those cultivating and processing the plant and naturally occurring contaminants such as microbes and fungi. The use of pesticides during cultivation is well established, but the validity of reports of a range of other adulterants in street cannabis, from oregano to cocaine, is less assured (McPartland and Pruitt, 1997).

Microbial contamination of cannabis exposes users to microbial toxins and possible infection by pathogenic organisms, including *Salmonella muenchen* (Taylor et al., 1982) *Thermactinomyces vulgaris*, *Micropolyspora faeni*, and *Thermoactinomyces candidus* (Kurup et al., 1983). These may not affect healthy individuals but in a review of medicinal cannabis use by immunocompromised patients such as those who have contracted HIV/AIDS or are undergoing cancer chemotherapy, McPartland and Pruitt concluded that microbiological contamination poses a serious risk to this patient group.

Cannabis plants can also be infected by many of the plant-pathogenic fungi which commonly cause opportunistic infections in immunosuppressed people, such as *Aspergillus flavus*, *Aspergillus fumigatus*, *Aspergillus niger*, *Penicillium chrysogenum*, *Penicillium italicum*, *Rhizopus stolonifer* and *Mucor hiemalis* (McPartland and Pruitt, 1997). It has been shown that spores of *Aspergillus fumigatus* survive in cannabis smoke (Kurup et al., 1983), carrying the risk of pulmonary aspergillosis.

Yet although a small cohort of AIDS patients with pulmonary aspergillosis found four out of six to be cannabis smokers (Denning et al., 1991), an uncontrolled clinical trial of 56 immunocompromised patients smoking cannabis did not report any cases of pulmonary infections (Vinciguerra et al., 1988), and no increased rate of opportunistic infections have been reported in an epidemiological study (Polen et al., 1993).

At least seven species of the *Fusarium* fungus infect cannabis plants (McPartland, 1991) and produce mycotoxins. One *Fusarium* toxin, zearalenone, causes a mycotoxicosis marked by nausea, vomiting, diarrhoea, headache, chills and convulsions (Rippon, 1988). *Alternarea alternata*, another fungus affecting cannabis, produces alteranariol, a mycotoxin which causes mutations in human esophageal epithelium, and may play an important role in cancer of the aerodigestive tract (Liu et al., 1992).

McPartland and Pruitt (1997) conclude that opportunistic fungi constitute the greatest hazard from cannabis for immunocompromised users, and they recommend sterilization of cannabis before smoking by heating in an oven at 150°C for five minutes.

Precautions for prescribing cannabinoids

Were cannabinoids to be prescribed as unlicensed medicines, it would be important for prescribing doctors to be aware of those conditions for which cannabinoids were contraindicated or where there were cautions against their use. For each cannabinoid, specific contraindications and cautions should be developed based on existing and further research. The risks that some cannabinoids could pose for patients with certain conditions would need to be balanced against the benefits. For instance, psychosis can be aggravated by some psychoactive cannabinoids, but research would be needed to ascertain whether a patient with mild psychosis and severe multiple sclerosis related pain could receive cannabinoid treatment beneficially. In addition, because THC can cause tachycardia (Vachon et al., 1976) the implications for patients with cardiovascular disease would need to be considered.

A doctor prescribing psychoactive cannabinoids has a duty of care to inform the patient of possible impairment of driving skills, machine operating, DIY etc and of additive effects with other sedative drugs including alcohol, benzodiazepines and opiates, and to record this advice in the patient's notes. The patient is then responsible for his actions and if found ignoring this advice and driving under the influence of such drugs, could be prosecuted under Section four of the Road Traffic Act 1988. It is not necessary for the patient to inform the Driver Vehicle Licensing Agency of their prescribed use of cannabinoids unless the condition for which they are being treated is itself notifiable.

Some of the psychological effects of psychoactive cannabinoids experienced by patients, particularly dysphoria and anxiety, could probably be minimised by preparation, explanation and reassurance given before the start of treatment. In addition, these effects may be partly prevented by co-administration of other drugs such as prochlorperazine, cannabidiol, or use of less psychoactive cannabinoids such as Δ^8-THC (see Nausea and vomiting associated with cancer chemotherapy, p.21-27). Intermittent courses rather than continuous treatment may limit the development of tolerance and prevent drug accumulation in cases where long-term therapy is required.

In view of the widespread use of cannabis for recreational purposes, it would be prudent to develop a labelling system that does not identify prescribed drugs as cannabinoids, and to warn patients that such drugs should be kept in a place inaccessible to others, especially children and adolescents.

5

Dosage and routes of administration

Optimal dosage and timing of administration has yet to be established for all indications. Routes of administration of cannabinoids also remain problematic. Anecdotal reports suggest that cannabis is more effective and has fewer unwanted effects when it is smoked than when it is taken orally (Grinspoon and Bakalar, 1993). This may be due to a number of factors. First, cannabis is much more rapidly absorbed when inhaled than when taken orally (see Pharmacokinetics, p.11-15). Secondly, other cannabinoids in cannabis smoke may enhance or modify the effects of THC. Thirdly, patients can exert a degree of control over the amounts of cannabinoids absorbed and hence over the nature and intensity of the symptoms they experience optimising the balance between beneficial and unpleasant effects. The health risks associated with smoking tobacco have been well documented, and many of the same constituents are present in cannabis smoke, including most of the known carcinogens (see Table 2). An increase in carboxyhaemoglobin as well as tar has also been described (Tau-Chin Wu et al., 1988). However, fully effective aerosol preparations of cannabinoids have yet to be developed, and research in this area is badly needed, so that cannabinoids can be administered quickly. Inhalation may also improve bio-availability in comparison with the oral route. Furthermore, if improved routes of administration are not developed, patients may resort to illegally smoking cannabis with the associated health and social risks.

When taken orally, cannabinoids are only slowly absorbed (see Pharmacokinetics, p.11-15). Furthermore, absorption is irregular and rates of first-pass metabolism in the liver vary greatly between individuals. However, the prolonged duration of effect may be therapeutically useful and merits further investigation. Administration of cannabinoids as rectal suppositories may be an alternative option. Cannabinoids are absorbed directly from the rectal mucosa, like those inhaled, and do not undergo first-pass metabolism from this site. Mattes et al. (1994) found that a rectal suppository, but not an oral capsule (both containing 2.5mg THC) increased appetite and food intake in normal subjects. The suppository also caused a greater increase in plasma THC than the capsule. Another possibility yet to be explored is the use of skin patches. Intravenous administration requires delivery as a fast-flowing saline infusion (see Pharmacokinetics, p.11-15) and is clearly not practical for long-term use.

6

Future prospects

Continuing basic research is likely to yield results that could greatly enhance the therapeutic potential of cannabinoids. The discovery of cannabinoid receptors makes possible the development of selective cannabinoid agonists and antagonists for use either as therapeutic agents or as experimental tools which may help to establish the physiological roles of cannabinoid receptors and of the endogenous compounds (anandamides) which bind to them. Such developments could lead to the synthesis of drugs with more specific actions than THC or nabilone or cannabis itself - e.g. cannabinoids with anti-emetic, analgesic or anticonvulsant effects without psychotropic or cardiovascular effects. Already there are some pointers in this direction: a selective and potent CB_1 antagonist (Rinaldi-Carmona et al., 1994) and two compounds that bind selectively to CB_2 receptors (Gareau et al., 1996) have recently been developed. Anandamides have not yet been tested in humans; it is possible that some of these might have specific actions on subtypes of cannabinoid receptors.

While cannabinoids penetrate the central nervous system, there are receptors present and some of the effects are clearly central, it is possible that some of the suspected therapeutic actions could be caused by action on peripheral tissue. These possible peripheral effects include vasodilatation, dry mouth, nausea relief, bronchodilatation, bladder effects and decrease of intraocular pressure. This possibility requires further pharmacological research because it is feasible that cannabinoids could be produced which do not penetrate the central nervous system and yet retain useful peripheral actions.

Meanwhile there is ample scope for further research on cannabinoids that have already been used in clinical trials. For example, Δ^8-THC appeared in one small trial to have excellent anti-emetic effects, without psychotropic actions, in children (Abrahamov et al., 1995). Further research with Δ^8-THC (which is cheaper to produce and more stable than THC: Mechoulam, personal communication) is merited for a range of illnesses including MS and other spastic conditions, and possibly asthma. In addition, cannabidiol appears to protect against the psychotropic effects of THC and further trials with this compound (and other non-psychoactive cannabinoids) used in combination with THC and nabilone should be encouraged.

Finally, some novel synthetic cannabinoids may turn out to have unexpected clinical uses. For example (+)-HU.210 (Table 1) has been shown to be a functional antagonist of NMDA (N-methyl-D-aspartate) receptors and may have uses in strokes, head injuries, and neurodegenerative disorders (Consroe and Sandyk, 1992).

7

Summary and recommendations

Arguments in favour of sanctioning cannabis for medical use have been based mainly on anecdotal reports (Grinspoon and Bakalar, 1993). Although many of these case histories sound convincing, and are often moving, they do not by themselves constitute scientific evidence (see Hall et al., 1994). On the other hand, the accumulation of scientific evidence has been hampered by regulations restricting the use of cannabinoids to one clinical indication (nabilone and dronabinol in the UK and dronabinol in the US as anti-emetics in cancer chemotherapy). It cannot be ignored that under these circumstances many normally law-abiding citizens - probably many thousands in the developed world - have resorted to the illegal use of cannabis to alleviate distressing symptoms inadequately controlled by existing drugs. Such therapeutic use should not be confused with recreational misuse.

This report has presented the information available from scientifically controlled trials of cannabis and cannabinoids in patients with various medical conditions, and related volunteer studies. The information is meagre but nevertheless it can be concluded that although cannabis itself is unsuitable for medical use, individual cannabinoids have a therapeutic potential in a number of medical conditions in which present drugs or other treatments are not fully adequate. Long-term effects of chronically

administered cannabinoids have not been studied, but present evidence indicates that they are remarkably safe drugs with a side-effects profile superior to many drugs used for the same indications.

There are two mechanisms by which the law could be changed in the UK to allow the prescription of those cannabinoids which are currently controlled under Schedule 1 of the Misuse of Drugs Act as having no medical use. The first involves the World Health Organization recommending to the United Nations Commission on Narcotic Drugs that certain cannabinoids should be rescheduled under the United Nations Convention on Psychotropic Substances so that they could be prescribed as a medicine. As a party to the convention, the UK Government would normally make a corresponding change to the misuse of drugs legislation to allow its prescription in the UK, (although under the terms of the Convention, countries are free to adopt stricter controls than those required by the Convention). This would be the responsibility of the Home Office.

Whilst this is the usual mechanism for affecting such changes, alternatively research-based evidence of the therapeutic benefits of cannabinol or other cannabinoids could be presented to the Home Office and Department of Health who could then consider modifying the Misuse of Drugs Act to allow their prescription by doctors.

The results of this review of research therefore leads the BMA to make the following recommendations:

1 The World Health Organization should advise the United Nations Commission on Narcotic Drugs to reschedule certain cannabinoids under the United Nations Convention on Psychotropic Substances, as in the case of dronabinol. In response the Home Office should alter the Misuse of Drugs Act accordingly.

2 In the absence of such action from the World Health Organization, the Government should consider changing the

Misuse of Drugs Act to allow the prescription of cannabinoids to patients with particular medical conditions that are not adequately controlled by existing treatments.

3 A central registry should be kept of patients prescribed cannabinoids so that the effects can be followed up over the long term.

4 The Clinical Cannabinoid Group,[2] interested patient groups, pharmaceutical companies and the Department of Health should work together to encourage properly conducted clinical trials to evaluate the further potential therapeutic uses of cannabinoids, alone or in combination, and/or in combination with other drugs.

5 The regulation of cannabis and cannabinoids should be sufficiently flexible to allow such compounds to be researched without a Misuse of Drugs Act licence issued by the Home Office.

6 Pharmaceutical companies should undertake basic laboratory investigations and develop novel cannabinoid analogues which may lead to new clinical uses.

7 To prevent misuse patients should be warned to keep these drugs in a place inaccessible to others.

8 In the absence of product licences, information similar to data sheets is required for all preparations of cannabinoids and equivalent compounds even if prepared from natural

2 The Clinical Cannabinoid Group is chaired by Dr Roger Pertwee. Its membership consists of those planning to set up clinical trials of cannabinoids and it aims to provide expertise, advice and knowledge to clinical researchers to facilitate such research. Contact: Dr Roger Pertwee, University of Aberdeen, tel. 01224 273040; e-mail rgp@aberdeen.ac.uk

substances. Standardised patient information should also be prepared after consultation with pharmacists.

9 Research on the clinical indications for medical prescription of cannabinoids should be undertaken. For all the indications listed below (i-vii) further research is required to establish suitable methods of administration, optimal dosage regimens and routes of administration.

i) *Anti-emetics*

Further research is needed on the use of Δ^8-THC as an anti-emetic, the use of cannabidiol in combination with THC, and the relative effectiveness of cannabinoids compared with 5-HT_3 antagonists. Further research is needed in other cases of nausea and vomiting such as post-operative.

ii) *MS, spinal cord injury and other spastic disorders*

A high priority should be given to carefully controlled trials of cannabinoids in patients with chronic spastic disorders which have not responded to other drugs are indicated. In the mean time there is a case for the extension of the indications for nabilone and THC for use in chronic spastic disorders unresponsive to standard drugs.

iii) *Pain*

The prescription of nabilone, THC and other cannabinoids (including the new more selective synthetic agents such as levonantradol, (-)-HU-210 and others in the process of development) should be permitted for patients with intractable pain. Further research is needed into the potential of cannabidiol as an analgesic in chronic, terminal and post-operative pain.

iv) *Epilepsy*

Trials with cannabidiol (which is non-psychoactive) used to enhance the activity of other drugs in cases not well controlled by other anticonvulsants are needed.

v) *Glaucoma, asthma*

Cannabinoids do not at present look promising for these indications, but much further basic and clinical research is needed to develop and investigate cannabinoids which lower intraocular pressure, preferably by topical application (eg eye drops; inhalant aerosols), without producing unacceptable systemic and central nervous system effects.

vi) *Stroke and neurodegenerative disorders*

The potential of (+)-HU-210 for these indications should be explored through further research.

vii) *Immunological effects*

Further research is needed to establish the suitability of cannabinoids for immunocompromised patients, such as those undergoing cancer chemotherapy or with HIV/AIDS.

10 Prescription formulations of cannabinoids or substances acting on the cannabinoid receptors should not include either cigarettes or herbal preparations with unknown concentrations of cannabinoids or other chemicals.

11 While research is underway, police, the courts and other prosecuting authorities should be aware of the medicinal reasons for the unlawful use of cannabis by those suffering from certain medical conditions for whom other drugs have proved ineffective.

Appendix I

Glossary

aerodigestive tract the upper part of the digestive tract which is shared with the respiratory system and is exposed to both air and food and includes the mouth, tongue, pharynx (throat) and nasal passages.

agonist an agent capable of stimulating a biological response by occupying cell receptors.

anorexia loss or absence of appetite for food.

anorexia nervosa aversion to food due to psychological causes, leading to severe weight loss.

antagonist an agent which opposes the action of another.

anti-emetic a drug which reduces the incidence and severity of nausea and vomiting.

antidyskinetic a drug which alleviates dyskinesia (the impairment of voluntary movements resulting in fragmented or jerky motions, as in Parkinson's disease).

antineoplastic preventing the development, maturation or spread of neoplastic (cancerous) cells.

anxiolytic a drug which reduces anxiety.

ataxia lack of balance and a tendency to fall when walking in the absence of paralysis.

autonomic (of the nervous system) the part of the nervous system which regulates the activities of blood vessels, secretory glands and organs and other soft inner parts of the body.

blood dyscrasia an abnormality of the blood or bone marrow.

bradycardia slow heart rate usually defined as less than 60 beats per minute in adults.

bronchoconstriction narrowing of the smaller bronchi and bronchioles (the smaller muscular air passages of the lungs).

bronchodilatation dilatation of the constricted small bronchi and bronchioles; the relaxation of a bronchoconstriction.

cachexia an extreme state of general ill health with malnutrition, wasting, anaemia and circulatory and muscle weakness.

cannabis (herbal) preparations of dried leaves, stalks, flowers, seeds from the plant *Cannabis sativa*; also known as marijuana or marihuana in the US.

cannabis resin resin secreted by the plants and prepared in blocks; also known as hashish.

cannabis oil product of extraction by organic solvents.

cannabinoids compounds which occur naturally only in the plant *Cannabis sativa* and some of its subspecies. The main plant cannabinoids are Δ^9-tetrahydrocannabinol (THC); Δ^8-tetrahydrocannabinol, cannabinol and cannabidiol. These all have a similar chemical structure, shown in Fig. 1. Synthetic cannabinoids, with differing chemical structures, include nabilone, levonantradol and others shown in Fig. 2. Anandamide is a natural substance found in animals which binds to cannabinoid receptors. It is sometimes referred to as an endogenous cannabinoid but has a different structure; it is a fatty acid derivative (arachidonyl ethanolanide) related to prostaglandins. Properties of various cannabinoids are summarised in Table 1.

conjunctival hyperaemia increase in the volume of blood in the conjunctiva due to arterial or arteriolar dilation. The increased volume of blood gives rise to reddening of the conjunctiva, a characteristic sign of recent cannabis use.

detrusor a muscle whose contraction results in expelling a substance.

drug tolerance a state of diminished responsiveness to a previously administered drug, so that a larger dose is required to produce the initial effect. Tolerance develops with repeated usage and may lead to lack of clinical effect, escalation of dosage and drug dependence.

drug dependence a state in which continued administration of the drug is required for psychological or physical well-being, and in which cessation of drug use (or decrease in accustomed dosage) results in withdrawal symptoms.

drug withdrawal syndrome (abstinence syndrome) a cluster of symptoms, psychological or physical or both, resulting from withdrawal of a drug on which a subject has become dependent. Withdrawal symptoms are usually unpleasant and are alleviated by a further dose of the drug, thus encouraging continued drug use. Withdrawal effects sometimes include rebound or "overshoot" effects, ie cannabinoids can reduce intraocular pressure (IOP) but sudden withdrawal may cause an increase in IOP above pre-treatment levels.

dyskinesia any abnormality of movement, such as incoordination, spasm or irregular and ill-formed movements.

dysphagia difficulty in swallowing.

dysphoria the condition of being ill at ease.

dyspnoea difficulty in breathing.

dystonia any abnormality of muscle tone.

extrapyramidal symptoms dystonias (cf) and dyskinesias (cf) arising from abnormalities in certain nuclei in the brain which contribute to muscle tone and movement but are anatomically distinct from the main motor system comprised of the pyramidal tracts passing from the brain to the spinal cord.

first-pass metabolism some orally administered drugs, including THC, after absorption from the gut, are partially or completely metabolised in their "first-pass" through the liver before reaching the general circulation. Blood concentrations do not therefore reach the same levels as those obtained by routes of administration (inhalation, sublingual, rectal) in which the drugs directly enter the circulation without first passing through the liver.

hepatotoxic destructive to liver cells.

hypokinesia reduced power of movement or motor function; slight paralysis.

hypotonia reduced tone or tension.

keratitis inflammation of the cornea.

myoclonic jerks a sudden shock-like muscular contraction which may involve one or more muscles or a few fibres of a muscle.

neuroleptic a drug that by its characteristic actions and effects is useful in the treatment of mental disorders, especially psychoses.

neuropathic pain pain resulting from damage to or destruction of nerve cells.

neurotransmitters/neuromodulators Endogenous (naturally occurring) agents which mediate or modulate the transmission of impulses in the nervous system. These include noradrenaline, dopamine, serotonin, acetyl choline, GABA (gamma aminobutyric acid), NMDA (N-methyl-D-aspartate), endogenous opioids and many others, probably including anandamide. All these substances exert their effects by binding to and interacting with one or more specific receptor.

nociceptive pain pain resulting from inflammatory reactions around the site of injury.

nocturia the need to urinate during normal sleeping hours.

nystagmus a condition in which the eyes are seen to move in a more or less rhythmical manner from side to side, up and down, or in a rotary manner from the original point of fixation which may result from one of several causes.

paraesthesia numbness and tingling.

parasympathomimetic a chemical agent that has a similar effect to the excitation of the parasympathetic nervous system, a subdivision of the autonomic nervous system (cf).

paroxysmal pain pain resulting from a sudden attack, as a convulsion or spasm.

photophobia an abnormal intolerance of light .

postherpetic neuralgia continuous neuralgic pain in an area previously the site of an attack of herpes zoster.

postural hypotension a condition in which the blood pressure falls when the person stands up.

psychic relating to the mind.

psychoactive the ability to alter mood, anxiety, behaviour, cognitive processes or mental tension.

psychological relating to the mind or mental processes.

psychotropic the ability to affect psychic function or behaviour.

psychotic affected by psychosis (those mental disorders which usually include organic mental disorder, the schizophrenias, major affective disorders and certain paranoid states).

receptors specific molecular sites in the body to which drugs (including cannabinoids) bind and through which they exert their effects. Cannabinoid receptors in humans include CB_1 receptors in the brain and CB_2 receptors in the spleen.

somnolence unnatural sleepiness or drowsiness.

supraspinal above the spine.

tachycardia rapid action of the heart, usually defined as rates exceeding 100 beats per minute in adults.

tardive dyskinesia a delayed dyskinesia (cf) consisting of extra-pyramidal symptoms (cf) caused by long-term exposure to neuroleptic drugs (cf).

thrombocytopenia a fewer than normal number of platelets per unit volume of blood. This can lead to poor blood coagulation and a risk of haemorrhage.

Tourette's syndrome a condition marked by repetitive, violent facial tics and incoordinated, purposeless, voluntary movement. Most cases involve the involuntary use of obscene words and spontaneous repetition of meaningless phrases.

Appendix II

Anecdotal evidence

To the clinical studies discussed in this report may be added numerous open trials and anecdotal reports of the beneficial effects of smoked cannabis. Below are some anecdotal accounts, which give an insight into particular patients' experiences, but which have not been subject to scientific evaluation. Case histories excerpted with permission from Yale University Press, Grimspoon L, Bakalar J B. (1993) *Marihuana, the Forbidden Medicine*. Yale University Press, New Haven and London and from Galen Press, Randall R C (ed.) (1991) *Muscle spasm, pain and marijuana therapy*. Galen Press, Washington DC.

Nausea and vomiting associated with cancer chemotherapy

Harris Taft was receiving chemotherapy for Hodgkin's disease. The account is given by his wife, Mona Taft.

> *One day in 1977, when we arrived at the treatment room where Harris was to receive the injection, he bolted and ran down the corridor. I found him a bit later, wandering the halls. He told me he couldn't take any more chemotherapy. He was at wit's end, exhausted by the disease, terrified by the effects of the drugs that were supposed to prolong his life. I have never before or since seen a man so genuinely and deeply frightened. Harris had come to fear the treatments more than the cancer and, he admitted, more than death itself. He told me he would choose dying over further chemotherapy.*

Later Harris tried smoking cannabis before chemotherapy; it completely controlled the vomiting.

> *It is impossible for me to adequately describe what a profound difference marihuana made. Before using marihuana, Harris felt ill all the time, could not eat, could not even stand the smell of food cooking. Afterward, he remained active, ate regular meals, and could be himself. His mood, his manner, and his overall outlook were transformed. And of course, marihuana prolonged his life by allowing him to continue chemotherapy. In two years of smoking it, he never had an adverse or untoward reaction. Marihuana was the least dangerous drug my husband received during the nine years he was treated for cancer.*

A second example is the well known science writer Professor Stephen Jay Gould who was treated for a mesothelioma.

> *I had surgery, followed by a month of radiation, chemotherapy, more surgery, and a subsequent year of additional chemotherapy. I found that I could control the less severe nausea of radiation by conventional medicines. But when I started intravenous chemotherapy (Adriamycin), absolutely nothing in the available arsenal of antiemetics worked at all. I was miserable and came to dread the frequent treatments with an almost perverse intensity.*
>
> *....[Smoking] marihuana worked like a charm. I disliked the "side effect" of mental blurring (the "main effect" for recreational users), but the sheer bliss of not experiencing nausea - and then not having to fear it for all the days intervening between treatments - was the greatest boost I received in all my year of treatment, and surely had a most important effect upon my eventual cure.*

(Grinspoon and Bakalar, 1993)

Pain from muscle spasticity in multiple sclerosis

Claire Hodges gives a typical description of the use of cannabis in MS for painful muscle spasms, bladder problems and other symptoms not well controlled by available medication:

> *I was being prescribed a whole range of medicines. There were pills to stop me feeling sick. There were pills to relieve bladder spasms but they made me feel sick and gave me blurred vision. There were pills to help me sleep but they made me anxious and were habit-forming....*
>
> *For about a year now, I have been regularly taking a small amount of cannabis resin - less than the size of half a pea - late at night. I used to smoke it.... but I was worried that my children might see me smoking so now I eat it. After a short time, my body completely relaxes, which relieves my tension and spasms. During the day I have to use a catheter whenever I want to empty my bladder and, most notably, cannabis relieves the discomfort and difficulty I have controlling it. It has also stopped the nausea that kept me awake at night.... I don't often take enough to "get high". When I do, I'm sure the feeling of calm and euphoria does my spirits a lot of good, too.*

(Hodges, 1993)

Spasms resulting from spinal injury

In 1969 David Brandstetter dived into the shallow end of a swimming pool and broke his neck. As a quadriplegic, having lost control over the movement of his arms and legs, he found cannabis to be an effective anti-spasmodic drug. The following extract is from his affidavit submitted before the US Drugs Enforcement Administration hearings *In the matter of marijuana rescheduling:*

> *...Upon leaving the hospital I was given a prescription for [diazepam] to reduce the severe spasms associated with my condition. During this time I developed a mild addiction to [diazepam]. While [diazepam] helped mask the spasms, it also made me more withdrawn and less able to take care of myself.*
>
> *I stopped taking [diazepam] because I feared the consequences of long-term addiction. However, my spasms became uncontrollable and were often so bad they would throw me out of my wheelchair.*
>
> *In 1973, I went to a party and someone offered me some marijuana, which I smoked. At the end of the party someone gave me some marijuana to take home.*
>
> *During this same period, I began going to a friend's house in the afternoons where we smoked marijuana. It was during this time that I noticed that the severe spasms stopped whenever I smoked marijuana.*
>
> *Unlike [diazepam], which only masked my symptoms and caused me to feel drunk and out of control, marijuana brought my spasmodic condition under control without impairing my facilities. In fact, marijuana actually enhanced my co-ordination. As a result, when I smoked marijuana regularly I was able to be more active. I did not have to constantly fight against the spasms. I became more active, alert, and outgoing. In addition to improving my limited muscle control, marijuana also improved my sense of wellbeing, which was critical to my recovery.*
>
> *Marijuana controlled my spasms so well that I could go out with friends and I began to play billiards again. The longer I smoked marijuana the more able I was to use my arms and hands. Marijuana also improved my bladder control and bowel movements.*

(Randall, 1991)

Glaucoma

Robert Randall had lost a substantial degree of vision due to glaucoma, his condition was worsening, and he had begun to smoke cannabis regularly. He gives the following account:

> *Despite my use of every pharmaceutical agent in the inventory, my evenings were routinely visited by tricolored halos - a signature of ocular pressures over 35 mm Hg [millimeters of mercury]. On some nights the halos were muted. On other evenings they appeared as hard crystal rings emanating from every source of light. And then there were nights, not so rare, of white-blindness - the world rendered invisible by its brilliance. Clinical translation: ocular tension in excess of 40 mm Hg. To summarize, things were not going very well.*
>
> *Then someone gave me a couple of joints. Sweet weed! That night I made and ate dinner, watched television. My tricolored halos arrived, which made watching TV less interesting. So I put on some good music, dimmed offending lights, and got into some serious toking. I happened to look out my window at a distant street lamp and noticed what was not there. No halos. That's when I had the full blown, omni-dimensional technicolor cartoon light-bulb experience. In a transcendent instant the spheres spoke! So simple. Old messages - new context. You smoke pot, your eye strain goes away.*

Robert Randall was under the care of Dr Ben Fine, an ocular pathologist.

> *...Doctor Fine, though mystified by the sudden change in my condition, was greatly pleased by the results. My ever-eroding visual fields stabilized. My slide into darkness slowed, then halted. As my glaucoma came under medical management, other aspects of life began to right themselves. I escaped welfare and took a part-time teaching job at a local college.*

(Grinspoon and Bakalar, 1993)

Epilepsy

Gordon Hanson, a 53 year old man, partially controlled his grand mal epilepsy and absence attacks with the standard drugs phenytoin, primidone, and phenobarbitone, but there were serious side effects.

> *Combinations of prescription drugs, including Dilantin, [primidone] and phenobarbital, did decrease the number of seizures but definitely did not cure the problems. Deep sadness would often overwhelm my life for days. Epilepsy was naturally assumed to be the cause - no one ever told me then that the drugs used to prevent seizures also had bad side effects.*

Experiencing marital and financial problems, Mr Hanson's seizures increased. A marriage counsellor suggested he might try cannabis to decrease the depressive effect of phenobarbital and still control the seizures.

> *...Thank God, I began to read about the plant and also made inquiries to other sources, including the University of Minnesota. I found out that it had been used medically in centuries gone by, and I began to smoke it regularly.*
>
> *By 1976 I cut my dose of phenobarbital, [phenytoin], and [primidione] by about 50 percent. Seizures had become less frequent and mood swings had dwindled, at least when marihuana was available.*

(Grinspoon and Bakalar, 1993)

Anorexia (Loss of appetite)

Ron Mason, was diagnosed with hepatitis B in 1983 and later with HIV. Following his diagnosis of hepatitis B, he found cannabis helpful in controlling his symptoms of nausea and vomiting:

Although I lacked appetite, the doctor told me I had to eat. Since I had a liver disease, I naturally gave up drinking (I had never drunk much anyway), and now began to smoke more marihuana. I noticed that my appetite increased dramatically after smoking. I began to smoke daily and gained weight rapidly. Two years later I had not yet produced antibodies and was officially designated a hepatitis carrier.

...In April 1984 I was referred by doctors at a gay VD clinic to what was later to become known as the AIDS clinic in Chicago. I saw doctors there for seven years and gained 40 pounds, achieving normal weight. The doctors knew I smoked marihuana and did not forbid it, although they urged moderation. I cannot tolerate AZT because of anemia. All the other antiviral drugs are damaging to my hepatitis-infected liver.

Three years ago one of my doctors told me that I am one of a handful of people who have been going to the clinic for several years and are not dead or gravely ill; the doctors don't know why. I attribute part of my success to smoking marihuana. It makes me feel as if I am living with AIDS rather than just existing. My appetite returns, and once I have eaten, I don't feel sick anymore. Marihuana improves my state of mind, and that makes me feel better physically.

(Grinspoon and Bakalar, 1993)

Migraine

Carol Miller, who suffers from migraine, describes her experiences as follows:

...it wasn't until college that I was given the diagnosis of migraine and received medication. The college infirmary prescribed [coated aspirin], which helped somewhat with the

> *headache but not with the visual effects or the nausea. It also gave me tremendous heart-burn.*
>
> *One time the pain was so severe that they gave me an injection of [a synthetic opioid], which pretty completely wiped out the pain but left me very lightheaded.*
>
> *...Several years later the migraines returned, and my husband said he had read that marihuana was good for headaches. I was amazed. Two hits and a short rest completely warded off the nausea and headache. As soon as I noticed flickering visuals that forewarned me of an approaching migraine, I could take a little cannabis and a short nap and the migraine would not develop at all. I was usually ready to go back to work in half an hour. It gave me a feeling of tremendous power to be finally in such control of my migraines.*
>
> *In the eighteen years since I began using cannabis to relieve migraines, I have been caught away from home several times without my herb. Once I tried taking Tylenol and found it helped a little with the pain but not at all with the nausea or the visual effects.*
>
> (Grinspoon and Bakalar, 1993)

Depression

The following patient gives her account of the effects of cannabis on her depression:

> *My first major episode of depression occurred in 1969, when I went away to college. I withdrew halfway through my freshman year and began semi-weekly therapy sessions with a psychiatrist. With her help and the use of a tricyclic antidepressant, I was able to return to a college closer to home the following September.*
>
> *...Under the guidance of these therapists I have tried more than a dozen different drugs, including several types of tricyclic anti-*

depressants, [fluoxetine], lithium, [methylphenidate, a stimulant related to amphetamine], synthetic thyroid hormone, and probably others I have forgotten. The only ones that have affected my moods significantly are [amitryptiline] at high doses and combinations of [dextroamphetamine] and a barbiturate. [Amitryptiline] works only during an incapacitating episode of depression, and its side effects, especially constipation, are distressing. Since use of [dextroamphetamine] and barbiturates as antidepressants is considered unorthodox, my therapist and I have been uneasy about it, but it was the only medication that worked. Several prominent psychiatrists have verified this and recommended that I use whatever helps. But now I am becoming tolerant to both of these drugs (I have been careful not to increase the dose, because I know the dangers).

In the spring of 1990 I smoked marihuana for the first time since 1973. To my amazement, a quarter of a joint changed my self-perception to match the person others saw. It was like night and day. I had experienced a similar change only a few times before, when [amitryptiline] kicked in and lifted me out of the depths. But with [amitryptiline] it took four days of rapidly increasing doses; with marihuana it took less than five minutes, every time. Since then I have been using marihuana to think clearly, to concentrate, and simply to enjoy the beauty of the world in a way I couldn't for years.

(Grinspoon and Bakalar, 1993)

Pain and spasms from rheumatoid arthritis

Lynn Hastings used cannabis to alleviate pain and spasms resulting from her rheumatoid arthritis. The following extract is from a sworn affidavit filed with the Court when she was tried for growing cannabis plants in 1989:

There is not any cure for my disease. I must do what I feel is right and safe for me. I want to live long enough to enjoy my grandchildren and have the most fulfilling life that I am able to have.

Marijuana has helped me very much. When I smoke a marijuana cigarette I receive instant relief from my pain. I am able to concentrate on my muscle spasms and relax the area that is giving me the most pain. The marijuana affects me like a wave of relief. The pain relief is fast and the effect on my mind is only for a couple of hours. I am able to think clearly without a drug hangover the next day.

The fatigue that I feel from my juvenile rheumatoid arthritis is also remedied within half an hour. I am able to do my housework or cook my family's dinner. I am able to talk to people and have a normal conversation with friends, family, or phone calls. Another benefit from the marijuana is that it helps me with my depression.

Depression is a minor factor to the pain, but the depression is more apparent with muscle relaxers and narcotics, the only other mode of pain relief that is available to me at this time. I am very concerned that I may become addicted to narcotics or that I will need to increase the narcotic in order to get the same relief that I am getting now. There are many people who have chronic pain that are addicted and need to increase their medication in order to obtain pain relief. Besides, I sleep much more on the narcotics than I did on marijuana.

I never felt that I needed the marijuana other than for pain and muscle spasm relief, nor did I need to increase the amount of marijuana to obtain the pain relief that I required.

(Randall, 1991)

Pain and other symptoms following brain surgery

Karen Ross gives the following account of the use of cannabis for the treatment of pain and other symptoms following brain surgery:

> *In 1988 I had surgery for a malignant brain tumor, an oligodendroglioma. The name is as overwhelming as the reality. Two days after the operation I read an article in the Boston Globe about the medical uses of marihuana, especially for people undergoing cancer treatments like radiation and chemotherapy. I had been a moderate user of marihuana before my catastrophic illness, and I took serious note of the article, since I was about to have radiation treatments.*
>
> *Within days after returning home I began to have severe anxiety attacks. Sometimes I thought I would lose my mind. I alternately felt as though my chest was going to burst open or be crushed. My hearing was so acute I could hear the bubbles inside a soda can. My speech was slurred, and I mixed up sounds so that people's words sounded like mumbles unless they were talking directly to me. Often I had to rely on lip reading. For these symptoms the doctor gave me [alprazolam], a tranquilizer, and [amitryptiline], an antidepressant. The medications helped somewhat, but I was still not comfortable.*
>
> *My family obtained some marihuana for me and I began to use it along with the Xanax and [amitryptiline]. I would smoke at most two "hits" a couple of times a day. I found that marihuana relaxed me and focused my attention, so that I felt less anxiety and rested more easily. It also relieved the pressure in my head better than dexamethasone. I did not experience a "high". I was already in emotional and physical overdrive, and the marihuana put me at cruising speed, regulated and even. Eventually I was able to reduce my use of Exines and stop using [amitryptiline] entirely.*

Six weeks after surgery I started taking radiation treatment and went on taking it five days a week for six weeks. Before and after each treatment I smoked marihuana. It allowed me to sleep during the treatment and took away the tightening and tingling sensation I would feel in my head afterward.

The dexamethasone caused me to gain sixty-five pounds. I also developed weakness in my muscles, especially in the knees, insomnia, mood swings, personality changes, potassium loss, and facial hair growth. When the dexamethasone was finally withdrawn, six weeks after the radiation treatments ended, I lost back most of the weight and regained most of my physical strength. My speech also became clearer (I still have a low tolerance for noise and still have to read lips to understand conversations).

All this time I continued to use marihuana. Eventually I returned to part-time work, but shortly afterward marihuana became unavailable. My headache pain, head and eye pressure, facial numbness, anxiety attacks, and slurred speech returned. A brain scan showed no changes in the tumor. When I managed to acquire some marihuana and smoke it, all the symptoms disappeared within a day. A couple of months later marihuana became unavailable again and my symptoms returned like clockwork.

(Grinspoon and Bakalar, 1993)

Appendix III

Summary of research studies

Table i: Selected well controlled studies on the antiemetic effects of THC in patients on cancer chemotherapy

Reference	Subjects	Drug and Dose
Sallan et al. (1975)	22 patients on cancer chemotherapy, resistant to standard drugs.	THC 10mg/m^2
Chang et al. (1979)	15 patients on high dose methotrexate.	THC 10mg/m^2 oral, 3 hrly 17mg smoking*
Frytak et al. (1979)	116 patients with gastrointestinal carcinoma on combined 5-fluouracil and semustine.	THC 15mg tds PCP 10mg tds
Orr and McKernan (1981)	55 patients on various cancer chemotherapy.	THC 7mg/m^2 qds PCP 7mg/m^2 qds
Lucas and Laszlo (1980)	53 patients on various cancer chemotherapy.	THC 15mg THC 5mg x 2 Standard antiemetics
Chang et al. (1981)	8 patients on adriamycin and cyclophosphamide.	THC 10mg/m^2 oral, 17.4mg smoking*, 3 hrly
Niedhart et al. (1981)	52 patients on various cancer chemotherapy.	THC haloperidol
Gralla et al. (1982)	27 patients on cisplatin.	THC 10mg/m^2 MCP 2mg/kg IV
Ungerleider et al. (1982)	214 patients on various cancer chemotherapy.	THC 7.5-12.5mg 4 hrly PCP 10mg 4 hrly
Lane et al. (1991)	62 patients on various cancer chemotherapy.	THC (dronabinol) 10mg qds PCP 10mg qds Both drugs together.

db - double blind; pc - placebo controlled; r - randomised; x - crossover; PCP - prochlorperazine; MCP - metoclopramide; tds - 3 times daily; qds - 4 times daily
* - THC smoked rather than taken orally if vomiting occurred

Type of study	Results
db, pc, r, x	THC significantly more effective than placebo for nausea and vomiting (patients' self-reports); sedation and euphoria on THC.
db, pc, r, x	14 of the 15 patients had decreased nausea and vomiting on THC compared with placebo.
db, pc	THC and PCP equally effective, both better than placebo. Side effects of THC sometimes intolerable - sedation, "high", dysphoria, hypotension, tachycardia.
db, pc, r, x	THC better than PCP, both better than placebo. THC produced "high" in 82%.
pc, r	THC more effective than standard regimes and placebo.
db, pc, r	THC ineffective compared with placebo.
db, pc, r, x	No difference between THC and haloperiodol in nausea and vomiting.
db, pc, r	MCP better than THC; both better than placebo for nausea and vomiting.
db, r, x	No significant difference between PCP and THC in control of nausea and vomiting; more side effects on THC but preferred by more patients.
db, r	No nausea and vomiting 51% for THC, 83% for PCP; PCP and THC combined better than either drug alone.

Table ii: Selected well-controlled studies on the antiemetic effects of nabilone in patients on cancer chemotherapy

Reference	Subjects	Drug and Dose
Nagy et al. (1978)	47 patients on cisplatin combination therapy.	Nabilone 2mg 6 hrly PCP 10mg 6 hrly
Herman et al. (1979)	113 patients on cisplatin, doxorubicin/cyclopho-sphamide, mustine.	Nabilone 2mg 6 or 8 hrly PCP 10mg 6 or 8 hrly
Einhorn et al. (1981)	100 patients on various cancer chemotherapy.	Nabilone 2mg 6 hrly PCP 10mg 6 hrly
Jones et al. (1982)	54 patients on various cancer chemotherapy.	Nabilone 2mg 6 hrly Placebo
Wada et al. (1982)	114 patients on various cancer chemotherapy.	Nabilone 2mg bd Placebo
Levitt (1982)	36 patients on various cancer chemotherapy.	Nabilone (dose not stated) Placebo
Johannson et al. (1982)	18 patients on various cancer chemotherapy.	Nabilone 2mg bd PCP 10mg bd
Ahmedzai et al. (1983)	26 patients with lung cancer on cyclophosphamide, adriamycin, and etoposide.	Nabilone 2mg bd PCP 10mg tds
Niiranan and Mattson (1985)	24 patients on various cancer chemotherapy.	Nabilone 2mg 6 hrly PCP 15mg 6 hrly
Niederle et al. (1986)	20 patients on cisplatin.	Nabilone 2mg 6 hrly Alizapride 150mg tds
Pomeroy et al. (1986)	38 patients on various cancer chemotherapy.	Nabilone 1mg 6 hrly Domperidone 20mg 6 hrly
Dalzell et al. (1986)	23 children on various cancer chemotherapy.	Nabilone 0.5-1mg bd or tds Domperidone 5-15mg tds
Chan et al. (1987)	30 children on various cancer chemotherapy.	Nabilone PCP

db - double blind; pc - placebo controlled; r - randomised; x - crossover;
PCP - prochlorperazine; bd = twice daily; tds = 3 times daily

Type of Study	Results
db, pc, r, x	Nabilone more effective than PCP or placebo for nausea and vomiting.
db, pc, r, x	Nabilone significantly more effective than PCP or placebo for nausea and vomiting.
db, r, x	Nabilone significantly more effective than PCP for nausea and vomiting, and preferred by 75% of patients. Lethargy and hypotension with nabilone.
db, pc, r, x	Significant reduction of nausea and vomiting with nabilone compared with placebo. Side effects common but acceptable (dizziness 65%; drowsiness 51%).
db, pc, r, x	Nabilone superior to placebo for nausea and vomiting. Side-effects frequent with nabilone but preferred by more patients.
db, pc, r, x	Nabilone superior to placebo for nausea and vomiting. Side-effects frequent but nabilone preferred by more patients.
db, r, x	Nabilone superior to PCP for nausea and vomiting. Nabilone preferred to PCP by patients, despite more side-effects.
db, r, x	Nabilone significantly more effective than PCP for nausea and vomiting. More side effects (drowsiness, dizziness) with nabilone but preferred by patients.
db, r, x	Nabilone significantly better than PCP for nausea and vomiting and preferred by most patients though more side effects.
db, r, x	Nabilone more effective than alizapride for nausea and vomiting, though more side-effects.
db, r	Nabilone significantly superior to domperidone for vomiting episodes.
db, r, x	Nabilone more effective than domperidone for nausea and vomiting though more side-effects. Two thirds of children preferred nabilone.
db, r, x	Nabilone was superior to PCP in nausea and vomiting.

Table iii: Studies on the effects of cannabis and cannabinoids in multiple sclerosis (MS)

Reference	Subjects	Drug and Dose
Petro and Ellenberger (1981)	9 patients with MS	Oral THC 5, 10mg, single doses.
Clifford (1983)	8 patients with MS	Oral THC 5-15mg 6 hourly, up to 18 hours.
Ungerleider et al. (1987)	13 patients with MS	Oral THC 2.5-15mg once or twice daily for 5 days.
Meinck et al. (1989)	1 patient with MS	Smoking cannabis, dose not stated, single dose.
Greenberg et al. (1995)	10 patients with MS 10 normal controls	Smoking cannabis. (1.54% THC) single dose.
Martyn et al. (1995)	1 patient with MS	Oral nabilone 1mg every second day for 2 periods of four weeks.
Consroe et al. (1996)	112 patients with MS in UK and USA	Smoking cannabis, dosage not known
Grinspoon & Bakalar (1993), Davies (1992), Doyle (1992), Ferriman (1993), Handscombe (1993), Hodges (1992, 1993), James (1993)	~10 patients with MS	Smoking or oral cannabis, dosage not known.

Type of study	Results
Double blind, placebo controlled	Significant reduction in objective spasticity scores overall after THC; one patient improved objectively after placebo, three patients subjectively improved, two of these objectively improved. Minimal psychoactive effects.
Single blind, placebo controlled	5 patients showed mild subjective but not objective improvement in tremor and well being after THC. 2 patients showed subjective and objective improvement in tremor, but not inataxia or other symptoms. All experienced a "high" after THC; 2 became dysphoric.
Double blind, placebo controlled	Significant subjective improvement in spasticity at doses of 7.5mg THC and above, but no change in objective measurements of weakness, spasticity, coordination, gait or reflexes. Side effects in 12 patients on THC and 5 patients on placebo.
Open trial	Improvement in tremor, spasticity and ataxia.
Double blind, placebo controlled	Cannabis impaired posture and balance in all subjects, causing greater impairment in MS patients. No other objective neurological changes but subjective improvement in some patients. "High" experienced with cannabis.
Double blind, placebo controlled	Improvement in general well-being, muscle spasms and frequency of nocturia with nabilone. Mild sedation but no euphoria with nabilone.
Questionnaire survey (48% response rate from 233 questionnaires)	Improvement in muscle spasms and pain, depression, tremor, anxiety, paraesthesiae, weakness, balance, constipation. No information on adverse effects.
Anecdotal reports	Increased well-being, improvement of walking, appetite, breathing, bladder control, and relief of muscle spasms.

Table iv: Studies on the effects of cannabis and cannabinoids in spinal cord injury and movement disorders

Reference	Subjects	Drug and Dose
Dunn and Davis (1974)	10 patients with a range of problems arising from spinal cord injury.	Cannabis
Petro (1980)	2 patients: 1 with spinal cord injury, 1 MS.	Cannabis
Malec et al. (1990)	24 patients with spinal cord injuries.	Cannabis
Maurer et al. (1990)	1 patient with spinal cord injury.	Oral THC 5mg, oral codeine 50mg, placebo, each given 18 times over 5 months.
Consroe et al. (1986)	5 patients with various dystonias.	Oral cannabidiol, 100-600mg/day over 6 weeks.
Sandyk and Awerbach (1988)	3 patients with Tourette's syndrome.	Cannabis smoking.
Frankel et al. (1990)	5 patients with Parkinson's disease.	Cannabis cigarette (2.9% THC) diazepam 5mg oral, levodopa/carbidopa (25mg/25mg) oral, apomorphine 1-5mg s.c. on consecutive days.
Consroe et al. (1991)	15 patients with Huntington's disease.	Oral cannabidiol 10mg/kg/day for 6 weeks.

Type of Study	Results
Patient survey of perceived effects	5/8 noted improvement in spasticity, 4/9 noted improvement in phantom limb pain, 1/9 noted worsening of bladder spasm and 2/10 worsening of urinary retention.
Open clinical report	Relief from pain and muscle spasms.
Questionnaire survey (53% response rate from 48 questionnaires)	21 of 24 who had used cannabis reported decrease in spasticity.
Double blind, placebo controlled	THC and codeine alleviated pain to a similar degree; THC had an additional beneficial effect on spasticity.
Open trial	20-50% improvement in dystonia, in all cases, but exacerbation of tremor and hypokinaesia in 2 patients with co-existing Parkinsonism.
Case reports	Alleviation of motor tics reported by patients; authors suggest that effects due to anxiolytic action of cannabis.
Open study	Improvement in tremor with levodopa and apomorphine; no improvement in any disability with cannabis or diazepam.
Double blind, placebo controlled	No beneficial effects.

Table v: Human studies on the analgesic effects of cannabis and cannabinoids

Reference	Subjects	Drug and Dose
Noyes et al. (1975a)	10 patients with cancer pain.	Oral THC 5, 10, 15, 20mg in random order
Noyes et al. (1975b)	36 patients with cancer pain.	Oral THC 10 and 20mg, oral codeine 60 and 120mg
Raft et al. (1977)	10 patients undergoing extraction of impacted molar teeth.	IV THC 0.22mg/kg and 0.44mg/kg, IV diazepam 0.157mg/kg
Petro (1980)	2 patients with painful muscle spasms (1 spinal cord injury, 1 MS).	Cannabis
Jain et al. (1981)	56 patients with postoperative pain.	IM levonantradol 1.5-3mg
Lindstrom et al. (1987) Cited by Consroe and Sandyk (1992)	10 patients with chronic neuropathic pain.	Oral cannabidiol 450mg/day in divided doses.
Maurer et al. (1990)	1 patient with spinal cord injury.	Oral THC 5mg, oral codeine 50mg, each given 18 times over 5 months.
Grinspoon and Bakalar (1993)	3 patients with various severe acute/chronic pain not controlled with opiates. 1 patient with migraine.	Smoking cannabis.

Type of Study	Results
Double blind, placebo controlled	Significant pain relief with 15 and 20mg THC compared to placebo. Drowsiness and mental clouding common.
Double blind, placebo controlled	THC 20mg and codeine 120mg gave equivalent and significant pain relief compared with placebo. THC caused sedation and mental clouding.
Double blind, placebo controlled	No analgesic effects of THC detected. Higher dose of THC was rated as least effective, diazepam most effective. 6 subjects preferred placebo to THC, 4 preferred low dose THC to placebo.
Open clinical report	Relief from pain and muscle spasms.
Double blind, placebo controlled	Significant pain relief with both doses of levonantradol compared with placebo. Drowsiness common with levonantradol.
Double blind, placebo controlled	No analgesic effect of cannabidiol compared to placebo. Sedation with cannabidiol in 7 patients.
Double blind, placebo controlled	THC and codeine alleviated pain to a similar degree; THC also relieved spasticity.
Anecdotal reports	Pain relief reported in all cases allowing reduction in other analgesics; no "high" reported.

Table vi: Human studies on the effects of THC in anorexia

Reference	Subjects	Drugs and Dose
Gross et al. (1983)	11 patients with primary anorexia nervosa.	Oral THC 7.5-30mg/day Diazepam 3-15mg/day for 2 weeks.
Plasse et al. (1991)	10 patients with AIDS-related diseases receiving anti-viral therapy.	Dronabinol (THC) 2.5mg tds "as needed" for 5 months.
Beale et al. (1995)	72 patients with AIDS-related illness.	Dronabinol (THC) 2.5mg bd Placebo for 6 weeks.

Table vii: Human studies on the effects of cannabis and cannabinoids in epilepsy

Reference	Subjects	Drug and Dose
Keeler and Reifter (1967)	1 patient with generalised epilepsy.	Smoking cannabis (7 occasions over 3 weeks).
Consroe et al. (1975)	1 patient with generalised epilepsy poorly controlled on standard drugs.	Smoking cannabis 2-5 times daily while continuing standard medication.
Cunha et al. (1980)	15 patients with generalised epilepsy poorly controlled on standard drugs; 16 healthy volunteers.	Oral cannabidiol 200-300mg/day vs. placebo added to standard therapy in patients. Oral cannabinol 3mg/kg/dy vs. placebo in controls. Treatment for 4.5 months in both patients and controls.
Ames and Cridland (1986)	12 epileptic patients not controlled on standard drugs.	Oral cannabidiol 200-300mg/day for 4 weeks.
Trembly et al. (1990) (Conference report cited by Consroe and Sandyk, 1992)	10 patients with generalised, focal or complex partial epilepsy, poorly controlled on standard drugs. 1 patient with epilepsy.	Oral cannabidiol 300mg/day for 6 months in addition to standard drugs. Oral cannabidiol 900-1200mg/day for 10 months.
Grinspoon and Bakalar (1993)	1 patient with complex partial seizures; 1 patient with generalised absence attacks.	Smoking cannabis.

Table vi *(cont.)*: Human studies on the effects of THC in anorexia

Type of Study	Results
Double blind, placebo controlled	No significant difference in weight gain between THC and diazepam. More side effects (dysphoria) with THC.
Open trial	Significant weight gain or reduction of weight loss compared to pre-treatment.
Double blind, placebo controlled	Significant reduction in nausea and weight loss, increased appetite and improved mood with THC compared to placebo.

Table vii *(cont.)*: Human studies on the effects of cannabis and cannabinoids in epilepsy

Type of Study	Results
Case report	Cannabis appeared to precipitate convulsions after a 6-month fit-free period without medication. Causal relationship not clear.
Case report	Unsatisfactory control on standard medication; no further fits while also smoking cannabis.
Double blind, placebo controlled	Cannabidiol improved control in 7 of 8 patients; 1 of 7 patients improved on placebo. Somnolence reported by 4 patients on cannabidiol. No psychotropic or neurological effects of cannabidiol noted in controls.
Double blind, placebo controlled	No significant effect of cannabidiol on seizure frequency.
Double blind, placebo controlled	No effect of cannabidiol on seizure pattern or frequency.
Open trial	Reduction of seizure frequency while on cannabidiol.
Anecdotal reports	Cannabis appeared to alleviate seizures in both patients.

Table viii: Human studies on the effects of cannabis and cannabinoids on intraocular pressure (IOP)

Reference	Subjects	Drug and Dose
Hepler and Frank (1971)	11 normal subjects	Smoking 2g marijuana (0.9% THC)
Hepler et al. (1976)	429 normal subjects	Smoking THC 1, 2 and 4% Oral THC 15, 30 and 40mg
	48 hospitalised patients	Smoking THC 1 and 2%
	11 patients with glaucoma	Smoking THC 1, 2 and 4% Oral THC 15mg
Perez-Reyes et al. (1976)	12 normal subjects	IV infusions of several cannabinoids
Cooler and Gregg (1977)	10 normal subjects	IV infusion of 1.5 or 3mg THC
Jones et al. (1981)	13 normal subjects	Oral THC 10-30mg 4 hourly
Grinspoon and Bakalar (1993)	Reports on 2 patients with glaucoma	Smoking and oral marijuana (dose not stated)
Merritt et al. (1980)	18 patients with glaucoma	Smoking THC 2%
Merritt et al. (1981)	8 patients with glaucoma and hypertension	eye drops (to one eye) 0.01%, 0.05%, 0.1% THC

Type of Study	Results
Open trial	9 of the 11 subjects had a 16-45% drop in IOP.
Double blind, placebo controlled	Dose related drop in IOP by about 30% for 2% THC.
Single blind, placebo controlled	Similar to above.
Open trial	7 patients responded as above, no effect in 4 patients.
Single blind, placebo controlled	Significant reductions in IOP with Δ^8-THC, Δ^9-THC, 11-OH-THC; little effect with cannabinol, cannabidiol, beta-OH-THC.
Double blind, placebo controlled	Reduction in IOP but increased anxiety and tachycardia.
Double blind, placebo controlled	Reduction in IOP but tolerance developed after 10 days; abrupt withdrawal caused rebound in IOP.
Anecdotal reports from mid-1970s	Alleviation of symptoms and reduction of IOP after failure of standard drugs: no information on type of glaucoma.
Double blind, placebo controlled	Significant reduction in IOP but hypotension, palpitations, and psychotropic effects.
Double blind, placebo controlled	Dose-related decrease in IOP in both eyes, mild hypotension with 0.1% THC, no psychotropic effects.

Table ix: Human studies on the effects of cannabis and cannabinoids in bronchial asthma

Reference	Subjects	Drugs and Dose
Tashkin et al. (1976)	14 asthmatic subjects	Smoked THC 2% Oral THC 15mg Isoprenaline 0.5% Placebo
Vachon et al. (1976)	17 asthmatic subjects	Smoked THC 0.9% and 1.9%
Williams et al. (1976)	10 asthmatic subjects	THC 200µg in metered dose inhaler. Salbutamol aerosol 100µg. Placebo
Tashkin et al. (1977)	5 asthmatic patients 11 normal volunteers	THC aerosol 5-20mg Smoked THC 2.2% Oral THC 20mg THC after 5 min Isoprenaline 125mg Placebo

Type of Study	Results
Double blind, placebo controlled	THC produced bronchodilatation nearly equivalent to isoprenaline. Smoked THC reversed experimentally induced bronchospasm.
Single blind	THC produced significant and prolonged bronchodilatation. Tachycardia noted at the higher dose.
Double blind, placebo controlled	THC and salbutamol significantly improved ventilation; onset quicker with salbutamol but both drugs equivalent at 1 hr.
Double blind, placebo controlled	THC effective as bronchodilator in normal subjects and 3 asthmatics. Effect of aerosol less than isoprenaline but significantly greater after 1-3 hrs. THC aerosol caused slight cough/chest discomfort in 3 control subjects, but moderate to severe bronchoconstriction with cough and chest discomfort in 2 asthmatics.

References

Abrahamov A, Abrahamov A, Mechoulam R. (1995) An efficient new cannabinoid anti-emetic in pediatric oncology. *Life Sciences*; **56**:2097-2102.

Adler MW, Geller EB. (1986) Ocular effects of cannabinoids. In: *Cannabinoids as therapeutic agents* (ed R Mechoulam) pp51-70, Boca Raton:CRC Press.

Agurell S, Halldin M, Lindgren J-E, Ohlson A, Widman M, Gillespie H, Hollister L. (1986) Pharmacokinetics and metabolism of Δ^1-tetrahydrocannabinol and other cannabinoids with emphasis on man. *Pharmacological Reviews*; **38**:21-43.

Ahmedzai S, Carlyle DL, Calder IT, Moran F. (1983) Anti-emetic efficacy and toxicity of nabilone, a synthetic cannabinoid, in lung cancer chemotherapy. *British Journal of Cancer*; **48**: 657-663.

Ames FR, Cridland S. (1986) Anticonvulsant effect of cannabidiol. *South African Medical Journal*; **69**:14.

Archer RA, Stark P, Lemberger L. (1986) Nabilone. In: *Cannabinoids as Therapeutic Agents* (ed R Mechoulam) pp 85-103, Boca Raton:CRC Press.

Beal JA, Olson R, Laubenstein L, Morales JO, Bellman P, Yangco B, Lefkowitz L, Plasse TF, Shepard KV. (1995) Dronabinol as a treatment for anorexia associated with weight loss in patients with AIDS. *Journal of Pain and Symptom Management*; **10**:89-97.

Beddow N. (1995) Personal communication from Multiple Sclerosis Self-help Groups.

Benewitz N L, Jones R T. (1981) Cardiovascular and metabolic considerations in prolonged cannabinoid administration in man. *Journal of Clinical Pharmacology*; **21**:214-223S.

Benson M, Bentley AM. (1995) Lung disease induced by drug addiction. *Thorax*; **50**:1125-11237.

Biezenek A. (1994) 'Pot' eased my daughter's pain. *BMA News Review*, March, 25

British Medical Association. (1997) *The Misuse of Drugs*. Amsterdam:Harwood Academic Publishers.

British Medical Association and the Royal Pharmaceutical Society of Great Britain. (1996) *British National Formulary, Number 32*. London:The British Medical Association and The Pharmaceutical Press.

British Thoracic Society, National Asthma Campaign et al. (1997) The British guidelines on asthma management 1995 review and position statement. *Thorax*; **52**:1-21S.

Cantwell R, Harrison G. (1996) Substance misuse in the severely mentally ill. *Advances in Psychiatric Treatment*; **2**:117-124.

Carlini EA, Cunha JM. (1981) Hypnotic and antiepileptic effects of cannabidiol. *Journal of Clinical Pharmacology*; **21**:417-427S.

Chan HSL, Correia JA, MacLeod SM. (1987) Nabilone versus prochlorperazine for control of cancer chemotherapy-induced emesis in children: a double-blind, crossover trial. *Pediatrics*; **79**:946-952.

Chang AE, Shiling DJ, Stillman RC, Godberg NH, Seipp CA, Barofsky I, Simon RM, Rosenberg SA. (1979) Delta-9-THC as an antiemetic in cancer patients receiving high-dose methotrexate. *Annals of Internal Medicine*; **91**:819-830.

Chang AE, Shiling DJ, Stillman RC, Goldberg NH, Seipp CA, Barofsky I, Rosenberg SA. (1981) A prospective evaluation of delta-9-tetrahydrocannabinol as an antiemetic in patients receiving adriamycin and cytoxan chemotherapy. *Cancer*; **47**:1746-1751.

Chesher GB, Jackson DM. (1985) The quasi-morphine withdrawal syndrome: effect of cannabinol, cannabidiol and tetrahydrocannabinol. *Pharmacology Biochemistry & Behavior*; **23**: 13-15.

Clifford DB. (1983) Tetrahydrocannabinol for tremor in multiple sclerosis. *Annals of Neurology*; **13**:669-671.

Consroe PF, Wood GC, Buchsbaum H. (1975) Anticonvulsant nature of marihuana smoking. *Journal of the American Medical Association*; **234**:306-307.

Consroe P, Snider R. (1986) Therapeutic potential of cannabinoids in neurological disorders. In: *Cannabinoids as Therapeutic Agents* (ed R Mechoulam) pp 21-49, Boca Raton:CRC Press.

Consroe P, Laguna J, Allender J, Snider S, Stern L, Sandyk R, Kennedy K, Schram K. (1991) Controlled clinical trial of cannabidiol in Huntington's Disease. *Pharmacology, Biochemistry & Behaviour*; **40**:701-708.

Consroe P, Sandyk R. (1992) Potential role of cannabinoids for therapy of neurological disorders. In: *Marijuana/Cannabinoids. Neurobiology and Neurophysiology* (eds Murphy L, Bartke A) pp 459-524, Boca Raton:CRC Press

Consroe P, Musty R, Tillery W, Pertwee RG. (1996) The perceived effects of cannabis smoking in patients with multiple sclerosis. *Proceedings of the International Cannabinoid Research Society*. P7.

Cooler P, Gregg JM. (1977) Effect of delta-9-tetrahydrocannabinol on intraocular pressure in humans. *Southern Medical Journal*; **70**:951-954.

Cunha JM, Carlini EA, Pereira E, Ramos OL, Pimentel C, Gagliardi R, Sanvito WL, Lander N, Mechoulam R. (1980) Chronic administration of cannabidiol to healthy volunteers and epileptic patients. *Pharmacology*; **21**:175-185.

Cunningham D, Bradley CJ, Forrest GJ, Hutcheon AW, Adams L, Sneddon M, Harding M, Kerr DJ, Soukop M, Kaye SB. (1988) A randomized trial of oral nabilone and prochlorperazine compared to intravenous metoclopramide and dexamethasone in the treatment of nausea and vomiting induced by chemotherapy regimens containing cisplatin or cisplatin analogues. *European Journal of Cancer and Clinical Oncology*; **24**:685-689.

Dalzell AM, Bartlett H, Lilleyman JS. (1986) Nabilone: an alternative antiemetic for cancer chemotherapy. *Archives of Diseases of Childhood*; **B9**:1314-19.

Davies C. (1992) Drug dealers saved my wife from her MS hell. *The Mail on Sunday*, 15th November.

Deadwyler SA, Hampson RE, Childers SR. (1995) Functional significance of cannabinoid receptors in brain. In: *Cannabinoid Receptors* pp 205-231. London:Academic Press.

Denning D W, Follansbee S E, Scolaro M et al. (1991) Pulmonary aspergillosis in the acquired immunodeficiency syndrome. *New England Journal of Medicine*; **324**:654-662.

Devane WA, Dysarz FA, Johnson MR, Melvin LS, Howlett AC. (1988) Determination and characterisation of a cannabinoid receptor in rat brain. *Molecular Pharmacology*; **34**: 605.

Devane W A, Hanus L, Breuer A, et al. (1992) Isolation and structure of a brain consitutent that binds to the cannabinoid receptor. *Science*; **258**:1946-9.

Doyle C. (1992) High, dry and happier. *The Daily Telegraph*, 24th November.

Prescribing unlicensed drugs or using drugs for unlicensed indications. (1992) *Drug and therapeutics bulletins*; **30**:97-99.

Dunn M, Davis R. (1974) The perceived effects of marijuana on spinal cord injured males. *Paraplegia*; **12**:175.

Einhorn LH, Nagy C, Furnas B, Williams SD. (1981) Nabilone: an effective antiemetic in patients receiving cancer chemotherapy. *Journal of Clinical Pharmacology*; **21**:64S-69S.

Evans F. (1991) The separation of central from peripheral effects on a structural basis. *Planta Medica* 1991; **57**:560-567.

Fabre LF, McLendon D. (1981) The efficacy and safety of nabilone (a synthetic cannabinoid) in the treatment of anxiety. *Journal of Clinical Pharmacology*; **21**:377S-382S.

Ferriman A. (1993) Marihuana: The best medicine? *The Times* 4th May 1993.

Finnegan-Ling D, Musty RE. (1994) Marinol and phantom limb pain: a case study. Proceedings of the International Cannabis Research Society 1994: p 53.

Formukong EA, Evans AT, Evans FJ. (1989) The medicinal use of cannabis and its constituents. *Phytotherapy Research*; **3**:219-231.

Frankel JP, Hughes A, Lees AJ, Stern GM. (1990) Marijuana for Parkinsonian tremor. *Journal of Neurology, Neurosurgery and Psychiatry*; **53**:436.

Frytak S, Moertel CG, O'Fallon JR, Rubin J, Creagan ET, O'Connell MJ, Schutt AJ, Schwartau NW. (1979) Delta-9-tetrahydrocannabinol as an antiemetic for patients receiving cancer chemotherapy. A comparison with prochlorperazine and a placebo. *Annals of Internal Medicine*; **91**, 825-830.

Gareau Y, Dufresne C, Gallant M, Rochette C, Sawyer N, Slipetz DM, Tremblay N, Weech PK, Metters KM, Labelloe M. (1996) Structure activity relationships of tetrahydrocannabinol analogues on human cannabinoid receptors. *Bioorganic & Medicinal Chemistry Letters*; **6**: 189-194.

Gold MS. (1991) Marijuana. In *Comprehensive Handbook of Alcohol and Drug Addiction.* pp 353-376. New York:Marcel Dekker Inc.

Gold MS. (1992) Marihuana and hashish. In *A Handbook of Drug and Alcohol Abuse. The Biological Aspects.* Chapter 7. (eds G Winger, FG Hofmann, JH Woods). pp117- 131. Oxford:Oxford University Press.

Gough T. (1991) *The Analysis of Drugs of Abuse*. Chichester:John Wiley & Sons.

Graham JDP. (1986) The bronchodilator action of cannabinoids. In: *Cannabinoids as therapeutic agents* (ed R Mechoulam) pp 147-158. Boca Raton:CRC Press.

Gralla RJ, Tyson LB, Clark RA, Bordin LA, Kelsen DP, Kalman LB. (1982) Antiemetic trials with high dose metoclopramide: superiority over THC, and preservartion of efficacy in subsequent chemotherapy courses. *Proceedings of ASCO Meeting* C-222.

Green K, Roth M. (1980) Marijuana in the medical management of glaucoma. *Perspectives in Opthalmology*; **4**:101-105.

Green K. (1982) Marijuana and the eye - a review. *Journal of Toxicology - Cutaneous and Ocular Toxicology*; **1**:3-32.

Green K, Roth M. (1982) Ocular effects of topical administration of Δ^9-tetrahydro-cannabinol in man. *Archives of Ophthalmology*; **100**: 265-267.

Greenberg HS, Werness SAS, Pugh JE, Andrus RO, Anderson DJ, Domino EA. (1994) Short-term effects of smoking marijuana on balance in patients with multiple sclerosis and normal volunteers. *Clinical Pharmacology & Therapeutics*; **55**: 324-328.

Grinspoon L, Bakalar JB. (1993) *Marihuana, the Forbidden Medicine.* New Haven and London:Yale University Press.

Gross H, Egbert MH, Faden VB, Godberg SC, Kaye WH, Caine ED, Hawks R, Zinberg N. (1983) A double-blind trial of delta-9-THC in primary anorexia nervosa. *Journal of Clinical Psychopharmacology*; **3**, 165-171.

Hall W, Solowij N, Lemon J. (eds) (1994) *The Health and Psychological Consequences of Cannabis Use* National Drug Strategy Monograph Series No 25, Canberra, Australian Government Publishing Service.

Handscombe M. (1993) Cannabis: why doctors want it to be legal. *The Independent*, 23rd February.

Harvey DJ. (1984) Chemistry, metabolism and pharmacokinetics of the cannabinoids. In *Marihuana in Science and Medicine* (ed GG Nahas) pp 37-108. New York:Raven Press.

Health Council of the Netherlands. Standing Committee on Medicine. (1996) *Marihuana as medicine*. Rijswijk: Health Council of the Netherlands, 21E.

Hepler RS, Frank IR. (1971) Marihuana smoking and intraocular pressure. *Journal of the American Medical Association*; **217**:1392.

Hepler RS, Frank IM, Petrus R. (1976) Ocular effects of marihuana smoking. In: *The Pharmacology of Marihuana* Volume 1 (ed MC Braude, S Szara) New York:Raven Press.

Herkenham M. (1995) Localization of cannabinoid receptors in brain and periphery. In *Cannabinoid Receptors* (ed R Pertwee) pp 145-166. London:Academic Press.

Herman TS, Einhorn LH, Jones SE, Nagy C, Chester AB, Dean JC, Furnas B, Williams ST, Leigh SA, Dorr RT, Moon TE. (1979) Superiority of nabilone over prochlorperazine as an antiemetic in patients receiving cancer chemotherapy. *New England Journal of Medicine*; **300**: 1295-1297.

Hodges C. (1992) Very alternative medicine. *The Spectator*, 1st August.

Hodges C. (1993) I wish I could get it at the chemist's. *The Independent*, 23rd February.

Hollister LE. (1986) Health aspects of cannabis. *Pharmacological Reviews*; **38**:1-20.

Hollister LE. (1988) Cannabis - 1988. *Acta Psychiatrica Scandinavica* Suppl 345; **78**:108-118.

Howlett AC, Bidaut-Russell M, Devane WA, Melvin LS, Johnson MR, Herkenham M. (1990) The cannabinoid receptor: biochemical, anatomical and behavioral characterisation. *Trends Neuroscience*; **13**: 420-423.

Ilaria RL, Thornby JI, Fann WE. (1981) Nabilone, a cannabinol derivative, in the treatment of anxiety neurosis. *Current Therapeutic Research*; **29**:943-949.

Jain AK, Ryan JR, McMahon FG, Smith G. (1981) Evaluation of intramuscular levonantradol and placebo in acute postoperative pain. *Journal of Clinical Pharmacol*; **21**:320S-326S.

James T. (1993) Breaking the law to beat MS. *The Yorkshire Post*, 27th September.

Jay WM, Green K. (1983) Multiple drop study of topically applied 1% Δ^9-tetrahydro-cannabinol in human eyes. *Archives of Ophthalmology*; **101**:591-594.

Johansson R, Kilkku P, Groenroos M. (1982) A double-blind, controlled trial of nabilone vs prochlorperazine for refractory emesis induced by cancer chemotherapy. *Cancer Treatment Reviews*; **9**, (Supplement B):25-33.

Johnson MR, Melvin LS. (1986) The discovery of nonclassical cannabinoid analgesics. In: *Cannabinoids as Therapeutic Agents* (ed R Mechoulam) pp 121-145. Boca Raton:CRC Press.

Jones RT, Benowitz N, Bachman J. (1976) Clinical studies of cannabis tolerance and dependence. In *Chronic Cannabis Use* (ed RL Dornbush, AM Freedman, M Fink). pp 221-239, New York:New York Academy of Sciences.

Jones RT, Benowitz N, Herning RI. (1981) Clinical relevance of cannabis tolerance and dependence. *Journal of Clinical Pharmacology*; **21**:143S-152S

Jones SE, Durant JR, Greco FA, Robertone A. (1982) A multi-institutional phase III study of nabilone vs placebo in chemotherapy-induced nausea and vomiting. *Cancer Treatment Review*; **9**:45S-48S.

Kaslow RA, Blackwelder WC, Ostrow DG, Yerg D, Pajenicek J, Coulson AH, Valdiserri RO (1989) No evidence for a role of alcohol or other psychoactive drugs in accelerating immunodeficiency in HIV-1-positive individuals. *Journal of the American Medical Association*; **261**:3424-3429.

Keeler MH, Reifler CB. (1967) Grand mal convulsions subsequent to marihuana use. *Diseases of the Nervous System*; **18**:474-475.

Kreutz DS, Axelrod J. (1973) Delta-9-Tetrahydrocannabinol: Localization in body fat. *Science*; **179**:391-392.

Kurup VP, Resnick A, Kagen SL et al. (1983) Allergenic fungi and actinomycetes in smoking materials and their health implications. *Mycopathologia*; **82**:61-64

Lal H, Bennett DA, Shearman GT, McCarten MD, Murphy R, Angeja A. (1981) Effectiveness of nantradol in blocking narcotic withdrawal signs through non-narcotic mechanisms. *Journal of Clinical Pharmacology*; **21**:361S-366S.

Lane M, Smith FE, Sullivan RA, Plasse TF. (1990) Dronabinol and prochlorperazine alone and in combination as antiemetic agents for cancer chemotherapy. *American Journal of Clinical Oncology*; **13**:480-484.

Lane M, Vogel CL, Ferguson J. (1991) Dronabinol and prochlorperazine in combination are better than either agent alone for treatment of chemotherapy-induced nausea and vomiting. *Proceedings of the American Society of Clinical Oncologists*; **8**:326.

Leirer VO, Yesavage JA, Morrow DG. (1991) *Aviation Space and Environmental Medicine*; **62**: 221-227.

Levitt M. (1982) Nabilone vs placebo in the treatment of chemotherapy-induced nausea and vomiting in cancer patients. *Cancer Treatment Reviews*; **9** (Supplement B):49- 53.

Levitt M. (1986) Cannabinoids as antiemetics in cancer chemotherapy. In: *Cannabinoids as Therapeutic Agents* (ed R Mechoulam) pp 71-83, Boca Raton:CRC Press.

Lindstrom P, Lindblom U, Boreus L. (1987) Lack of effect of cannabidiol in sustained neuropathia. Paper presented at Marijuana '87 Int. Conf. on Cannabis, Melbourne, September 2 to 4, 1987. (cited by Consroe & Sandyk, 1992).

Liu G Y, Qian P, Zhang W, Dong Y Q, Guo H. (1992) Etiological role of Alternaria alternata in human esophageal cancer. *China Medical Journal*; 1992; **105**:394-400.

Lucas VS Jr, Lazlo J. (1980) Δ^9-THC for refractory vomiting induced by cancer chemotherapy. *Journal of the American Medical Association*; **243**:1241-1243.

Malec J, Harvey RF, Cayner JJ. (1982) Cannabis effect on spasticity in spinal cord injury. *Archives of Physical and Medical Rehabilitation*; **63**:116-118.

Martyn CN, Illis LS, Thom J. (1995) Nabilone in the treatment of multiple sclerosis. *Lancet*; **345**:579.

Matsuda LA, Lolait SJ, Brownstein MJ, Young AC, Bonner TI. (1990) Structure of cannabinoid receptor and functional expression of the cloned DNA. *Nature*; **346**: 561.

Mattes RD, Engelman K, Shaw LM, Elsohly MA. (1994) Cannabinoids and appetite stimulation. *Pharmacology Biochemistry and Behavior*; **49**:187-195.

Maurer M, Henn V, Dittrich A, Hofmann A. (1990) Delta-9-tetrahydrocannabinol shows antispastic and analgesic effects in a single case double-blind trial. *European Archives of Psychiatry and Clinical Neuroscience*; **240**:1-4.

Maykut MO. (1985) Health consequences of acute and chronic marihuana use. *Progress in Neuro-Psychopharmacology & Biological Psychiatry*; **9**:209-238.

McPartland J M. (1991) Common names for diseases of Cannabis sativa L. *Plant Diseases*; **75**:226-227.

McPartland J M, Pruitt P L. (1997) Medical marijuana and its uses by the immuno-compromised. *Alternative Therapies*; **3**:39-45.

Mechoulam R. (1973) Cannabinoid chemistry. In: *Marijuana - Chemistry, Pharmacology, Metabolism and Clinical Effects* (ed R Mechoulam) pp1-99, London: Academic Press.

Mechoulam R. (1986) The pharmacohistory of cannabis sativa. In: *Cannabinoids as Therapeutic Agents* (ed R Mechoulam) pp 1-19, Boca Raton:CRC Press Inc.

Meinck HM, Schönle PW, Conrad B. (1989) Effect of cannabinoids on spasticity and ataxia in multiple sclerosis. *Journal of Neurology*; **236**:120-122.

Mendelson JH. (1987) Marihuana. In: *Psychopharmacology: The Third Generation of Progress* (ed HY Melter), pp1565-1571, Raven Press: New York.

Merritt JC, Crawford WJ, Alexander PC, Anduze AL, Gelbart SS. (1980) Effect of marijuana on intraocular and blood pressure in glaucoma. *Ophthalmology*; **87**:222-228.

Merritt JC, Olsen JL, Armstrong JR, McKinnon SM. (1981) Topical Δ^9-tetrahydrocannabinol in hypertensive glaucomas. *Journal of Pharmacy & Pharmacology*; **33**: 40-41.

Meuser K T, Yarnold P R, Levinson D F I, Singh H, Bellack A S, Kee K, Morrison R L, Yadalam K G. (1990) Prevalence of substance abuse in schizophrenics demographic and clinical correlates. *Schizophrenia Bulletin*; **16**:31-56.

Munro S, Thomas KL, Abu-Shaar M. (1993) Molecular characterization of peripheral receptor for cannabinoids. *Nature*; **365**:61-65.

Musty RE, Reggio P, Consroe P. (1995) A review of recent advances in cannabinoid research and the 1994 international symposium on cannabis and the cannabinoids. *Life Sciences;* **56**: 1933-40.

Nagy CM, Furnas BE, Einhorn LH, Bond WH. (1978) Nabilone: antiemetic crossover study in cancer chemotherapy patients. *Proceedings of the American Society for Cancer Research;* **19**: 30.

Nahas GG. (1975) Marihuana: toxicity and tolerance. In: *Medical Aspects of Drug Abuse.* (ed RW Richter) pp 16-36, Maryland:Harper & Row.

Nahas GG. (1984) The medical use of cannabis. In: *Marihuana in Science and Medicine* (ed Nahas GG) pp 247-261, New York:Raven Press.

National Institutes of Health. (1995) *Asthma Management and Prevention. A Practical Guide for Public Health Officials.*National Institutes of Health:USA

Negrete J C, Knapp W P, Duglas D E, Smith W B. (1986) Cannabis affects the severity of schizophrenic symptoms: results of a clinical survey. *Psychological Medicine;* **16**:515-520.

Niederle N, Schutte J, Schmidt CG (1986) Crossover comparison of the antiemetic efficacy of nabilone and alizapride in patients with nonseminomatous testicular cancer receiving cisplatin therapy. *Klinische Wochenschrift;* **64**:362-365.

Niedhart J, Gagen M, Wilson H, Young D. (1981) Comparative trial of the antiemetic effects of THC and haloperidol. *J Clin Pharmacol;* **21**:38S.

Niiranen A, Mattson K. (1985) A cross-over comparison of nabilone and prochlorperazine for emesis induced by cancer chemotherapy. *American Journal of Clinical Oncology;* **8**:336-340.

Noyes R, Brunk SF, Baram DA, Baram A. (1975a) Analgesic effect of delta-9-tetrahydro-cannabinol. *Journal of Clinical Pharmacology;* **15**:139-143.

Noyes R, Brunk SF, Baram DA, Canter A. (1975b) The analgesic properties of delta-9-THC and codeine. *Clinical Pharmacology & Therapeutics;* **18**:84-89.

Orr LE, McKernan JF. (1981) Antiemetic effect of delta-9-THC in chemotherapy-associated nausea and emesis as compared to placebo and compazine. *Journal of Clinical Pharmacology;* **21**:76S-80S.

Paton WDM, Pertwee RG. (1973) The actions of cannabis in man. In *Marijuana: Chemistry, Pharmacology, Metabolism and Clinical Effects* (eds GG Nahas and WDM Paton), pp 735-738, Oxford:Pergamon Press.

Perez-Reyes M, Wagner D, Wall ME, Davis KH. (1976) Intravenous administration of cannabinoids and intraocular pressure. In: *The Pharmacology of Marihuana* (eds MC Braude, S Szara); pp 829-32, New York:Raven Press.

Pertwee RG. (1990) The central neuropharmacology of psychotropic cannabinoids. In: *Psychotropic Drugs of Abuse* (ed Balfour DJK) pp 355-429, New York:Pergamon Press.

Pertwee RG. (1991) Tolerance to and dependence on psychotropic cannabinoids. In: *The Biological Bases of Drug Tolerance and Dependence* (ed Pratt JA). pp 231-263, London: Academic Press.

Pertwee RG. (1995) Pharmacological, physiological and clinical implications of the discovery of cannabinoid receptors: an overview. In: *Cannabinoid Receptors* (ed Pertwee RG) pp 1-34. London:Academic Press.

Petro DJ. (1980) Marihuana as a therapeutic agent for muscle spasm or spasticity. *Psychosomatics*; **21**:81-85.

Petro DJ, Ellenberger C. (1981) Treatment of human spasticity with Δ^9- tetrahydrocannabinol. *Journal of Clinical Pharmacology*; **21**:413S-416S.

Plasse TF, Gorter RW, Krasnow SH, Lane M, Shepard KV, Wadleigh RG. (1991) Recent clinical experience with dronabinol. *Pharmacology Biochemistry & Behavior*; **40**:695- 700.

Polen M R, Sidney S, Tekawa I S, Sadler M, Friedman G D (1993) Health care use by frequent marijuana smokers who do not smoke tobacco. *Western Journal of Medicine*; **158**:596-601.

Pomeroy M, Fennelly JJ, Towers M. (1986) Prospective randomized double-blind trial of nabilone versus domperidone in the treatment of cytotoxic-induced emesis. *Cancer Chemotherapy & Pharmacology*; **17**:285-288.

Prescribing unlicensed drugs or using drugs for unlicensed indications (1992). *Drug and therapeutics bulletin*; **30**:97-99.

Raft D, Gregg J, Ghia J, Harris L. (1977) Effects of intravenous tetrahydrocannabinol on experimental and surgical pain. Psychological correlates of the analgesic response *Clinical Pharmacology and Therapeutics*; **21**, 26-33.

Randall R C (ed) (1991) *Muscle spasm, pain and marijuana therapy*. Galen Press: Washington DC.

Razdan RK, Howes JF, Pars HG. (1983) Development of orally active cannabinoids for the treatment of glaucoma. In: *Problems of Drug Dependence* (ed Harris LS) pp 157-163. NIDA Research Monograph 43. Department of Health and Human Services: Washington DC.

Regelson W, Butler JR, Schulz J, Kirk T, Peek L, Green ML, Zalis MO (1976) Delta-9-THC as an effective antidepressant and appetite-stimulating agent in advanced cancer patients. In: *The Pharmacology of Marihuana* (eds MC Braude, S Szara); pp 763-776, New York:Raven Press.

Rinaldi-Carmona M, Barth F, Héaulme M, Shire D, Calandra B, Congy C, Martinez S, Maruani J, Néliat G, Caput D, Ferrara P, Soubrié P, Brelière KC, Le Fur G. (1994) SR141716A, a potent and selective antagonist of the brain cannabinoid receptor. *FEBS Letters*; **350**:240-244.

Rippon J W. (1988) *Medical Mycology.*3rd ed Philadelphia:Saunders.

Sallan S, Zinberg N, Frei E III. (1975) Antiemetic effect of delta-9-tetrahydrocannabinol in patients receiving cancer chemotherapy. *New England Journal of Medicine*; **293**:795-7.

Sandyk R, Awerbuch G. (1988) Marijuana and Tourette's syndrome. *Journal of Clinical Psychopharmacology*; 8:444.

Schwartz RH, Voth EA. (1995) Marijuana as medicine: making a silk purse out of a sow's ear. *Journal of Addictive Diseases* **14**:15-21.

Segal M. (1986) Cannabinoids and analgesia. In: *Cannabinoids as therapeutic agents* (ed R Mechoulam) pp 105-120; Boca Raton:CRC Press.

Stephens RS, Roffman RA, Simpson EE. (1993) Adult marijuana users seeking treatment. *Journal of Consulting and Clinical Psychology*; **61**:1100-1104.

Tashkin DP, Shapiro BJ, Frank IM. (1976) Acute effects of marihuana on airway dynamics in spontaneous and experimentally produced bronchial asthma. In: *The Pharmacology of Marihuana* (eds MC Braude, S Szara), New York:Raven Press.

Tashkin DP, Reiss S, Shapiro BJ, Calvarese B, Olsen JL, Lodge JW. (1977) Bronchial effects of aerosolized Δ^9-tetrahydrocannabinol in healthy and asthmatic subjects. *American Review of Respiratory Disease*; **115**:57-65.

Taylor D N, Wachsmuth I K, Shangkuan Y-H, et al. (1982) Salmonellosis associated with marijuana. *New England Journal of Medicine*; **306**:1249-1253.

Trembly B, Sherman M. (1990) Double-blind clinical study of cannabidiol as a secondary anticonvulsant. Paper presented at Marijuana '90 In. Conf. on Cannabis and Cannabinoids, Kolympari (Crete), July 8 to 11, 1990. (cited by Consroe & Sandyk, 1992)

Twycross RG, McQuay HJ. (1989) Opioids. In: *Textbook of Pain* (eds PD Wall, R Melzack). 2nd Edition, pp 686-701. London:Churchill Livingstone.

Ungerleider JT, Andrysiak T, Fairbanks L, Goodnight J, Sarna G, Jamison K. (1982) Cannabis and cancer chemotherapy. A comparison of oral delta-9-THC and prochlorperazine. *Cancer*; **50**: 636-645.

Ungerleider JT, Andrysiak T, Fairbanks L, Ellison GW, Myers LW. (1988) Delta-9-THC in the treatment of spasticity associated with multiple sclerosis. *Advances in Alcoholism and Substance Abuse*; **7**:39-50.

Vachon L, Mikus P, Morrissey W, FitzGerald M, Gaenser E. (1976) Bronchial effects of marihuana smoke in asthma. In: *The Pharmacology of Marihuana* (eds MC Braude, S Szara); pp 777-784, Raven Press: New York.

Vincent BJ, McQuiston DJ, Einhorn LH, Nagy CM, Brames MJ. (1983) Review of cannabinoids and their antiemetic effectiveness. *Drugs*; **25** (Suppl. 1): 52-62.

Vinciguerra V, Moore T, Brennan E. (1988) Inhalation marijuana as an antiemetic for cancer chemotherapy. *New York State Journal of Medicine*; **88**:525-527.

Wada JK, Bogdon DL, Gunnell JC, Hum GJ, Gota CH, Rieth TE. (1982) Double-blind, randomized, crossover trial of nabilone vs placebo in cancer chemotherapy. *Cancer Treatment Reviews*; **9** (Supplement B):39-44.

Williams SJ, Hartley JPR, Graham JDP. (1976) Bronchodilator effect of delta-9-THC administered by aerosol to asthmatic patients. *Thorax*; **31**: 720-723.

Wu TC, Tashkin DP, Djaheb B, Rose JE. (1988) Pulmonary hazards of smoking marijuana as compared with tobacco. *New England Journal of Medicine*; **31**:347-51.

Index